DRGs:
Changes
and Challenges

Franklin A. Shaffer, RN, EdD
Editor

Pub. No. 20-1959

National League for Nursing • New York

CONTENTS

Part III

PREFACE

When the Social Security Amendments of 1983 ushered in the era of prospective payment for hospitalization on a national level, those of us who had worked with the system in the State of New Jersey since the 1970s were surprised only at the speed with which the action took place. With the increase in health care costs—at a level much higher than that of the GNP—and the threat of bankruptcy to the Social Security system and in particular to the Medicare trust fund, it was obvious that some remedy must be found.

The tying of prospective payment to diagnosis related groups (DRGs) seems, at this point, to be only the first step in a process that will totally change the health care scene. There will, without doubt, be many modifications in the system of prospective payment—in the regulations that govern it, if not in the legislation itself. Already mandated are studies to evaluate and reassess the system and its outcomes.

Nevertheless, for now DRGs are a very present reality, one that affects not only every health care provider in an acute-care setting, but potentially all others as well. Although this publication focuses on the acute-care settings now under Medicare prospective payment, we would be remiss not to point out that some health industry analysts believe that the greatest impact of DRGs will ultimately be on home health care agencies. The Health Care Financing Agency has commissioned a five-year study aimed at developing prospective payment alternatives for home health. The impact of hospital prospective payment on the home health sector is already becoming evident—patients presenting themselves for home care are more acutely ill, have needs for higher levels of care, and require some complex treatments. It remains to be seen just what type of payment system will develop in this area.

Nurses, as the providers who spend more time with patients than any other and as the providers who document more care-related data than any other, are directly affected by the DRG system. Therefore, it is urgent that nurses understand as much as possible about DRGs and the prospective payment system that implements them. This book is an attempt to provide a source for that understanding. Written for nurses, with the concerns and activities of nurses in mind, the papers in this volume were prepared by nurses and other specialists who have dealt with the various challenges presented by the conversion to this new system. Several of the papers included were originally published in the pages of *Nursing & Health Care*, NLN's official journal.

The changes resulting from the shift to prospective payment have indeed presented us all with terrific challenges. To the extent that we can meet these challenges with positive and creative action, nurses can lead the way, in the name of a double concern—for professionalism and for the patient—to more effective and more efficient health care for all.

Franklin A. Shaffer, RN, EdD

FOREWORD

In designing prospective payment, we took several factors into account. First was the hospital inflation rate, which was running triple that of the rest of the economy. The total bill for health care in the United States was $322 billion in 1982, amounting to a tab of $1,400 for every man, woman, and child in America. This year Americans will turn 11 percent of the gross national product over to the health care industry.

Secondly, we were equally concerned about the status of the Medicare trust fund. Our actuaries had predicted that if we did nothing, the trust fund would be insolvent by 1990. In order to guarantee continued access to health services for Medicare beneficiaries, we knew that we had to slow down outlays.

These facts indicated some serious structural deficiencies in the old payment system. It was clear to us that in restructuring that system for greater efficiency, we also had to design incentives to restructure behavior patterns. I believe that in general the health care community understood the necessity for behavior change, and we had widespread cooperation in implementing prospective payment.

Under the old reasonable cost reimbursement system, essentially we had what I call the "open checkbook" phenomenon. All health care services deemed medically necessary were simply paid for after the fact. There is no inherent incentive in that type of system for better management. In effect, we invited increases in the length of stay and the number of ancillary tests.

We know from historical experience that we can track what the average cost would be for an average case in any of the 468 diagnosis related groups that are defined in the prospective payment system. We are now saying that we will pay a prudent buyer's fair price for these services. This clearly provides a cost-containment incentive, because we are telling management to operate within a specific budget.

For the first time, we have defined 468 product lines, and that product is the direct patient care that is given to a patient. In order to track their costs on a very accurate product line level, hospitals are, for the first time, setting in motion computerized programs to merge their clinical and financial data. This will enable them to determine how much it costs to care for a patient with a given disease entity on a given unit and enable comparative analysis that will promote more management efficiency. There are incentives in the system to identify nursing costs specifically, which I believe will eventually lead to much more autonomy and self-control for nursing.

Under prospective payment, the patient care component must be managed in such a fashion so as not to increase length of stay. It seems to me that the nurse who is at the bedside 24 hours a day is in the best position to accurately assess and monitor the patient's condition, and to intervene if necessary in order to prevent the kind of complications that can prolong normal length of stay.

Equally important is the nurse's role as patient coordinator, which is vital to keeping the length of stay manageable and to the kinds of therapeutic teaching plans that need to be done to assist in an early discharge and placement program. Accurate coordination of the whole spectrum of care from the time the patient comes into the hospital can shave at least a day off length of stay.

These roles, crucial to the success of prospective payment, are unique to nursing. The challenge to the health care system today is linking quality and cost efficiency, which the nurse is in a pivotal position to accomplish.

Carolyne K. Davis, RN, PhD
Administrator, Health Care Financing Administration

THE GROUND FOR CHANGE: MEDICARE

Franklin A. Shaffer

The speed with which the new prospective payment legislation was passed by Congress in April 1983 was remarkable and attributable to two major factors, at once political and financial: the increasing federal deficits and the threatened insolvency of the Medicare trust fund. Since the system for prospective payment is laid on the foundation of Medicare, one must have a basic understanding of the Medicare program as a background to understanding the workings of prospective payment.

The prospective payment system based on diagnosis related groups (DRGs) applies initially only to Medicare, the federally financed health insurance program for the aged, and not to payments by private insurers or by individuals who pick up the whole tab for their hospitalizations. However, since the federal government, through Medicare, is the nation's largest purchaser of health care, what happens in Medicare is a good indication of what will happen in the entire industry. Therefore, the system of prospective reimbursement for Medicare, especially if successful in containing health care costs, will probably spread throughout the health care system.

For the benefit of nurse managers who have not worked directly with federally financed health insurance, this introduction to Medicare will serve to summarize its provisions. (Care in other than the acute-care hospital is included to give a fuller picture.)

THE ENABLING LEGISLATION

The Medicare provisions for support of the medical expenses of our country's elderly were enacted into law in 1965 as Title XVIII of the Social Security

1

Act. Medicare (and its companion for the indigent, Medicaid, which was enacted as Title XIX of the Social Security Act) is administered by the Health Care Financing Administration (HCFA) of the U.S Department of Health and Human Services. Although it has been amended several times in its 19-year history—most recently and most pertinent to this discussion by the Tax Equity and Fiscal Responsibility Act (TEFRA) of 1982 (P.L. 97-248) and the Social Security Amendments of 1983—the original Medicare system retains the basic form outlined in the following paragraphs.

THE BENEFICIARIES OF MEDICARE

Anyone over 65 years of age is eligible for Medicare, and eligibility begins on the first day of the month when an individual turns 65. (At present, policy analysts concerned about the solvency of the Medicare trust fund are discussing increasing the age for eligibility.) Medicare is also available to certain disabled people under the age of 65 who have received Social Security benefits for 24 consecutive months and to people with end-stage renal disease, if they are currently entitled to Social Security benefits or if they are the spouses or dependent children of insured persons.

MEDICARE BENEFITS

The Medicare program is separated into two components: Part A, which is *hospital insurance*; and Part B, which is *medical insurance*. Claims and payments under Medicare are handled, not directly by the government itself, but by private insurance organizations under contract with the government. Insurance organizations handling claims for Part A, hospital insurance, are called *intermediaries;* those handling claims for Part B, medical insurance, are called *carriers.*

Medicare is introduced to its beneficiaries in the government's pamphlet, *Your Medicare Handbook* (January 1984), with the following caveat: "Under the law, Medicare does not cover custodial care or care that is not 'reasonable and necessary' for the diagnosis or treatment of an illness or injury." Each of these concepts is difficult to define absolutely, and even more difficult to enforce. Utilization review and peer review, as well as review by the insurance carrier, are the chief agents for evaluating "reasonable and necessary" charges. Apart from these restrictions, Medicare insures its beneficiaries against the cost of treatment of illness and injury as completely as most private insurance plans and more completely than many.

Part A Benefits

What is called Medicare hospital insurance actually includes payments toward care in a skilled nursing facility, home health care, or hospice, with unique provisions for each.

In a *hospital* participating in Medicare, the major services covered for an inpatient are:

—a semiprivate room

—all meals, including special diets

—regular nursing services

—costs of special care units

—drugs furnished by the hospital during the stay unless deemed less than effective

—blood transfusions except for the first three pints

—lab tests included in the hospital bill

—x-rays and other radiology services billed by the hospital

—such supplies as casts, surgical dressings, splints

—use of wheelchairs and other appliances

—operating and recovery room costs, including hospital costs for anesthesia services

—rehabilitation services

Medicare pays for 90 days of hospital care in each benefit period. A "benefit period" measures the time from admission to a hospital (or other health care facility) until the time of discharge; after 60 consecutive days out of the hospital, a new benefit period begins. An extra 60 days of eligibility, called the reserve days, may be used only once at whatever time or times the beneficiary chooses.

If emergency treatment is received in a hospital that doesn't participate in Medicare or if a nonparticipating hospital alone is equipped to handle an emergency, Medicare will honor the bill. In participating psychiatric and tuberculosis hospitals, Medicare will make payment for no more than 190 days in a lifetime.

In a *skilled nursing facility*, Medicare will pay for up to 100 days of care in each benefit period when the following conditions are fulfilled: (1) the beneficiary was a hospital inpatient for three successive days before the transfer, (2) the beneficiary was transferred for the condition that was treated in the hospital or for a related condition, (3) the beneficiary was admitted within 30 days after leaving the hospital, (4) a doctor certifies that skilled nursing or skilled rehabilitation services are needed daily and skilled services are received daily, and (5) the facility's utilization review committee approves the stay. HCFA is studying the probable cost of dropping the three-day hospitalization requirement, as mandated by TEFRA, but the outlook appears negative.

Similar to provisions for hospital care, Medicare covers a semiprivate room, regular nursing services, rehabilitative services, blood (after the first three pints), drugs, medical supplies and appliances. Medicare will not pay for custodial care only, for care in a skilled nursing facility occasionally, or for rehabilitative services that are no longer improving the condition of the patient.

As to cost-sharing for skilled nursing care, the beneficiary pays nothing for the first 20 days and $44.50 per day for days 21 to 100.

Home health care is payable under Medicare for patients who meet these conditions: (1) patient requires part-time skilled nuring care, physical therapy, or speech therapy, (2) need is certified by a doctor who plans the home care, (3) patient is confined to the house, and (4) services are provided by a certified home health agency.

If a patient requires skilled nursing care, physical therapy, or speech therapy, Medicare would then also pay for occupational therapy, part-time services of home health aides, medical social services, and medical supplies *except drugs* and equipment provided by the home health agency.

Beneficiaries of home health care are not required to share costs, and there is no time limit on home care deemed medically necessary.

Fewer than a million of the 13.5 million individuals enrolled in **health maintenance organizations** (HMOs) are Medicare or Medicaid beneficiaries. This results from a federal policy that has strongly encouraged the development of HMOs, but has not heretofore supported this choice of a health insurance plan for Medicare beneficiaries. (This will soon change with the implementation of a provision of TEFRA.) Congress has authorized HMOs and competetive medical plans (CMPs) to contract with Medicare beneficiaries on a prospective, per-capita basis for reimbursement at 95 percent of the rate that Medicare pays fee-for-service practitioners.

HMOs and CMPs must provide at least the minimum package of Medicare services, and the plans must prove their own solvency by means that still await federal regulations. There is some evidence that the competitive HMOs and CMPs will offer more than the minimum Medicare package, including vision, dental, and home health services.

Hospice, the treatment facility most recently permitted to participate in Medicare, was authorized by TEFRA for a three-year trial period beginning November 1, 1983. It carries the difficult-to-define stipulation that Medicare hospital insurance will be allowed for beneficiaries *whose life expectancy is six months or less.* Medicare will pay for a maximum of seven months of hospice care. If a patient still needs hospice services after this period is exhausted, the hospice must continue care unless the patient no longer wants its services.

Other conditions for Medicare reimbursement are that the patient has chosen to receive care from the hospice and that the hospice program is certified by Medicare. Medicare pays the full cost for the following services: nursing services; doctor's services when the doctor is employed by the hospice; drugs for pain relief and symptom management; physical therapy, occupational therapy, and speech/language pathology; home health aide and homemaker services; medical social services; medical supplies and appliances; and counseling. Medicare pays all but five percent of the cost of inpatient respite care, which is an inpatient stay of no more than five days in a row to give relief to the person who regularly assists in the home care. Part B of Medicare will contribute toward the charges of a patient's personal physician.

Part B Benefits

"Necessary and reasonable" medical and related services are covered by Medicare Part B. Whether a doctor's charge is reasonable is determined by the insurance carrier, who looks at the doctor's customary charges for the service, the prevailing charge for that service in the region, and what seems reasonable to a medical review committee. The carrier will approve the lowest of the three charges (actual, customary, or prevailing), and Medicare will pay 80 percent of the charge approved by the carrier. Where the charge is not approved, the patient is responsible for paying any remainder, plus the regular copayment of 20 percent of the bill and an annual deductible of $75.

A doctor may agree to accept the charge the carrier determines is reasonable, under an arrangement known as "assignment." If doctor and patient agree to the assignment method, then the doctor will receive payment directly from Medicare and not charge the patient the 20 percent copayment.

The Social Security Act contains a provision that Medicare beneficiaries may not be held liable for charges that they could not reasonably have been expected to know were not covered by Medicare. Providers, too, are paid for ineligible service when they could not have known payment would be denied.

Reimbursable doctors' services may be given in the home, office, hospital, or other recognized treatment facility (such as a renal dialysis center) and may include: drugs and biologicals that a patient can't administer to himself (insulin is excluded); diagnostic tests and procedures, including tests performed within seven days of hospital admission; and medical supplies and certain prosthetic devices. Excluded from payment are routine examinations, cosmetic surgery, and eye or hearing examinations for the purpose of prescribing eyeglasses or hearing aids.

Other related services accepted by Medicare are: physical therapy under the direction of a physician; major dental work, such as surgery of the jaw; an optometrist's examinations for aphakia; speech and physical therapy provided in a doctor's office or a hospital or approved agency; and manipulation by a chiropractor to correct subluxation that has been demonstrated by x-ray.

Charges for Medical Care in Hospitals

Reasonable charges for medical care in hospitals will be paid by Medicare Part B, if the doctor has personally performed the service and if the service must normally be performed by a doctor. If the doctor and hospital have drawn up a formal agreement on allocation of time, then a portion of the reasonable cost will be paid under Medicare Part A.

TEFRA has changed payments for medical care in hospital outpatient departments, which was once the same as for care in a doctor's office, to avoid paying for hospital overhead twice. Medical care in a hospital outpatient department will now be reimbursed under Part B at 60 percent of the prevailing rate for services in offices. Radiologists will be reimbursed at 40 percent of the prevailing rate.

THE FINANCING OF MEDICARE

Part A of Medicare, hospital insurance, is financed primarily through a tax on earnings under the Social Security Act and secondarily by proceeds from the railroad retirement fund and interest on funds deposited with the U.S. Treasury.

Beneficiaries share in the cost through a *deductible* and *coinsurance*. For hospital care, a deductible of $356 is required for the first 60 days, and the beneficiary is required to pay $89 a day coinsurance for days 61 to 90. In addition, for the one-time, nonrenewable 60 reserve days of hospital care, a coinsurance of $178 daily is required. After that time, for any single continuous hospital stay, Medicare pays nothing.

A quarter of Part B of Medicare (medical insurance) is financed by the payment of a premium of $14.50 a month by Medicare beneficiaries. This premium is raised each January 1 to approximately a quarter of the total cost for Part B insurance. The remainder comes from general revenues and from interest on funds deposited with the Treasury. As well as a premium, beneficiaries pay an annual deductible of $75 and 20 percent of "reasonable" charges.

Very needy Medicare recipients may be assisted by Medicaid, a joint state-federal insurance program for providing health care to the poor. Under this plan, states pay the premium for Medicare Part B insurance and the deductive and copayment for both Parts A and B. Medicare is unique to each state and benefits differ among the states. HCFA has proposed that each state have the option of whether or not to pay the Medicare deductible and coinsurance.

THE PROVIDERS AND MEDICARE

Hospitals and other health care facilities must meet state and local requirements and Medicare's conditions of participation in order to be reimbursed under Medicare. Only in the instance of necessary emergency treatment is the rule waived.

Medicare's conditions of participation for a hospital are met when a hospital is accredited by the Joint Commission on the Accreditation of Hospitals or the American Osteopathic Association. Certain hospitals that do not seek accreditation, such as small rural hospitals, are inspected by state health agencies following HCFA guidelines. At present, the following are required of a hospital: governing body, medical staff, nursing services, medical records, pharmaceutical services, radiological services, laboratory services, food and dietetic services, utilization review, physical environment, medical library. Optional services are outpatient, emergency, and social services. Skilled nursing facilities and home health agencies are accredited for Medicare participation by state agencies following federal guidelines.

Reimbursement for Nurses

The question of third-party reimbursement for nurses came to the forefront of health policy discussions with the enactment of the Rural Health Clinics Act on November 30, 1977. This legislation provided payment, for the first time, for nurse practitioner services to clinics in rural, underserved areas. The major features of the bill included:

—Reimbursement under Medicare at 80% of reasonable cost;

—Reimbursement under Medicaid at 100% of reasonable cost.

The services were to be provided under a physician's standing orders, but the physician did not have to be present.

The major problem with the legislation from nursing's standpoint was that the bill applied only to states with no statutory prohibitions against independent practice by nurse practitioners. There were, and are currently, in many states outright prohibitions against acts of diagnosis and prescription by any provider other than the physician.

SUMMARY

As inflation struck the health care industry, the fiscal problems of the Medicare trust fund created a crisis situation where reform was mandatory. The result was the system of prospective payment for Medicare that is the subject of the rest of this book.

THE CHALLENGE:
HEALTH CARE IN CRISIS

Pamela J. Maraldo

Unacceptably high health costs are old news by now. Health care costs are still escalating at a more rapid pace than the rest of the economy; the consumer price index for all goods and services lies at 4-5%, whereas the health care index for inflation still is around 11-12%. A recent Harris Poll tells us that everybody is dissatisfied with health care costs except physicians. In Washington, health programs are built around the theme of survival: how to cut costs and still provide quality; how to cut costs and set priorities; how to survive in a cutback management environment. Understandably, a feeling of apprehension is pervasive among health care professionals.

Everything has taken a back seat to the economy—environmental issues, women's issues, civil rights—topics prominent for the past ten years or so have all but disappeared. This is because economic recovery has been the overriding goal of lawmakers in this country. We used to ask for money for nurse training, and Congress was extremely willing to "help the girls out." But in the area of legislation, there has been a dramatic departure from business as usual. Since Ronald Reagan took office, most bills have been passed in accordance with strict spending ceilings for the first time in history. We have even seen cutbacks in the once sacrosanct Medicare program. Under the Reagan administration, there is no question that the country has moved further away from the goal of providing a common health security base for the poor and disadvantaged.

Since taking office, the Reaganites have not managed all the changes they sought in the health care economy; for instance, they did not manage to cap Medicaid. But for the most part, they have been tremendously successful, certainly more successful than health and social welfare advocates have been in bringing down military spending.

9

Nevertheless, the cutbacks in health care have clearly been a bipartisan effort. No matter who is in the White House, the drive to cut health and social welfare programs will press on, since over half of the federal budget is still spent on health and social welfare programs. Both parties have supported substantial budget cuts in the health area, with the end result that health care, as we have known it in this country, is gone.

The enactment of two major pieces of legislation under Reagan initiated the very substantial policy changes we have now. These laws were the Tax Equity and Fiscal Responsibility Act (TEFRA) and the Omnibus Reconciliation Act of 1982. The greatest hardships suffered by the health field so far were the consequences of these laws and the resulting cuts in the nation's two largest health programs: Medicare and Medicaid. These two programs account for the largest single portion of health care spending. Changes in these programs have great implications for all other aspects of health care. Inasmuch as Medicare and Medicaid account for over 10% of the total federal budget and their expenditures have been increasing at the rate of 20% per year, these programs were particularly vulnerable to the budget axe.

Major changes legislated by TEFRA and the Omnibus Reconciliation Act were:

—*Limits on reimbursement to hospitals:* Routine operating costs were limited to 108% of the mean, and the costs of ancillary services (laboratory, special care units, x-rays and blood tests) were also limited.

—*Three-year target rate:* Each hospital will have a target for increased Medicare cost-per-admission based on the previous year's allowable cost per case, increased according to the hospital's wage and price index.

—*Increase in coinsurance*

—*Increase in Part B deductible:* From $60.00 to $75.00

—*Elimination of the 5% nursing salary cost differential.*

In addition, twenty health and social services categorical programs were lumped together into four large block grants and tranferred to state and local governments. The four blocks became: (1) prevention; (2) primary care; (3) maternal child health; and (4) mental health, alcohol, and drug abuse. These changes altered the nature of health care responsibility and availablity in very fundamental ways.

Every single actor in the health care arena has been affected seriously. First, the patients or consumers who have been conspicuously absent from the dialogue. Medicare and Medicaid recipients will be affected in many ways. Individuals who no longer receive AFDC, CETA, food stamps, welfare, or who are unemployed, will be unable to pay for medical expenses. Hospital occupancy rates have dropped to around 65% nationally since the recession began in 1981 and have yet to recover. That fact, coupled with the cutbacks in payments to hospitals which have thus been less able to extend charitable care, has created a situation that is rather horrendous. With inflation and a high rate of unemployment, patients have been less able to afford hospitals, and hospitals less able to afford patients who cannot pay. The closing of a number of community health centers has meant a greater patient influx to outpatient departments in hospitals as well. (In outpatient departments, where patients used to have to wait four or five hours to see a provider, they now have to wait 11 to 12 hours—if they see a provider at all.)

In a situation of this nature, a hospital has had two choices. One is to shift the expenses from patients who cannot pay to patients who can—cost shifting to private patients. Or it can refuse to accept patients who cannot afford to pay. Both options have been widely practiced. Many public hospitals and clinics—those with the largest charity caseloads—have been unable to cope with the increased load of indigent patients and, with no hope of government subsidies, have been forced to close.

Hospitals serving middle-class populations have been better able to stay financially solvent because private patients, generally those with commerical hospitalization insurance, subsidize the care rendered to patients in Medicare and Medicaid programs. Thus, six billion dollars in costs were shifted in 1983.

Even given the increasingly critical nature of this situation, the initial cutbacks were considered to be superficial, and were not considered to hold much promise for salvaging the Medicare trust fund. Therefore, the Secretary of HHS was mandated under the terms of TEFRA to develop *a prospective payment proposal* for hospital care.

THE WHIRLWIND PASSAGE OF PROSPECTIVE PAYMENT

Just about everyone who was watching prospective payment travel through Congress was extremely surprised by the speed with which the proposal was passed—especially considering the notorious strength of the hospital lobby. But the crisis nature of the situation made it apparent that it was either do something quickly or watch the Medicare trust fund evaporate. So in three short months H.R.-1900 became law.

When the administration first sat down to develop a prospective payment proposal, as mandated in TEFRA, they had to decide how, out of all the different ways prospective payment could be calculated, they were going to approach the situation. Prospective payment can be calculated by case (AHA plan), by day (the method currently used in the cost-based scheme), or by patient (the capitation method that has generally been used by HMOs). The administration finally decided on *payments by type of diagnosis* because they believed this method would give hospitals the fewest opportunities to take advantage of the system. Health care people are highly disturbed by this choice because grouping hospital resource use by diagnosis does not take severity of illness into consideration. The apparent and simple logic of the method overrode objections, however, and the ultimately desired result of uniformity of payments won the day. The point of this method is that patients with similar diagnoses use similar amounts of resources. Why, it was asked, should a patient pay $2,100 to have a hip replaced in one state and $8,200 in another, when the procedures are virtually the same?

Birth of the Proposal

In the plan originally outlined by HHS Secretary Schweiker, the federal government would pay all hospitals the same basic amount, fixed in advance, for treating any patient with a particular diagnosis. Basic payments would be indexed to inflation, taking into account regional variations in wages and the costs of other goods and services. This amounted to a bare-bones approach to containing hospital costs. The plan included neither a quality review program nor any adjustments based on the size or location of a hospital. There was simply one flat national rate per DRG for every hospital in the country.

Significant changes were made during congressional deliberations that gave hospitals somewhat more flexibility and leeway, but not as much as they would have liked. Congressional debate centered around (1) whether DRG rate calculations would be based more on the individual hospital experience (AHA position) or on an aggregate, flat national rate for all hospitals (basically, the end result was a compromise); and (2) whether hositals would be able to bill patients the difference between what Medicare pays and what it will actually cost the hospital to deliver the service. Hospitals argued that physicians are permitted to do this under Medicare Part B, and that they (the hospitals) should have the same privilege. But there was no compromise here, and the House leadership strongly opposed any further increase in beneficiary payments.

Some concessions were made in favor of individual hospitals, but by and large the essence of the administration's original proposal remained intact. The finished product was approved by a conference committee of the House and Senate on March 25, 1983. Despite several amendments that will make it easier for hospitals to live in the new world of DRGs, prospective payment will dramatically change the nature of the health care delivery system as we know it today.

THE SOCIAL SECURITY ACT AMENDMENT OF 1983 PROSPECTIVE PAYMENTS FOR MEDICARE INPATIENT HOSPITAL SERVICES

Effective Date/Transition. Transition to the prospective payment system will begin on the hospital's first accounting period on or after October 1, 1983. Implementation of the prospective payment system will be phased in over a three-year period. In the first year, 25% of the payment will be based on regional DRG rates, and a 75% weighting will be based on the hospital's historic cost experience. In year two, 50% of the payment will be based on a blend of national and regional DRG rates (25% national, 75% regional); 50% of the payment will be based on each hospital's last experience. In year three, 75% of the payment will be based on a blend of national and regional DRG rates (50% national, 50% regional); 25% of the payment will be based on each hospital's cost experience. In year four, 100% of the payment would be based upon national DRG rates.

Payment Provisions. The national DRG-based prospective payment system will apply only to Medicare and not to all third-party payors. Amounts will be adjusted for rural and urban hospitals within nine census regions. Hospitals will keep payment amounts in excess of costs and absorb any costs in excess of DRG rates. Hospitals will not be permitted to charge co-payments and deductibles in excess of amounts now required by law. Rates will be based on historical cost data and the annual industry-wide increase in hospital costs. Rates will be updated in FY84 and FY85 using an index of the costs of goods and services purchased by hospitals plus one percentage point. In subsequent years, rates of DRG increases will be based on the opinion of a commission of experts.

Capital Costs. Capital-related costs will be excluded from the prospective rate. For the first three years of implementation, capital costs other than return on equity will be reimbursed on a reasonable-cost basis. For the first three years return on equity will be reimbursed at the same rate as the average interest rate on the Medicare Hospital Insurance Trust Fund, which is down one and one-half times from the current rate. Beginning after October 1, 1986, all capital costs, including return on equity, will be prospectively reimbursed.

Educational Costs. Direct teaching costs—including the costs of nursing education programs—would continue to be paid on a reasonable-cost basis and would be excluded from the prospective payment determinations. Indirect teaching expenses would be reimbursed at twice the amount of the teaching adjustment under TEFRA.

Quality Review. Hospitals would be required to contract with professional review organizations to review the quality of care provided, the appropriateness of Medicare admissions and appropriateness of care to patients designated as outliers.

Alternative Cost Control Systems. The Secretary of Health and Human Services can permit alternative cost control systems if it does not result in greater Medicare expenditures above what the government would otherwise have paid. Other criteria would have to be met at the discretion of the Secretary.

Exceptions and Exclusions. Psychiatric, long-term care, children's, and rehabilitation hospitals will continue to be reimbursed under the cost-based system.

Physician Reimbursement. The Secretary would be required to collect data and to report to Congress on the advisability and feasibility of including physician payments in DRG rates.

DRGs:
HISTORY AND OVERVIEW

Franklin A. Shaffer

On April 20, 1983, President Reagan signed into law H.R. 1900 (P.L. 98-21), the Social Security Amendments of 1983. This legislation includes the establishment of a prospective payment system based on 467 Diagnosis Related Group (DRG) categories that allow pretreatment diagnosis billing categories for almost all United States hospitals reimbursed by Medicare. Culminating a series of hospital billing and reimbursement reforms that were initiated decades ago, these changes will permanently alter the nature of health care delivery as we have known it.

The decades of latency characterizing the early history of this reform contrast sharply with its sudden explosive arrival. The entire legislative process, from submission before Congress to passage into law, took only an unprecedented three months. While the looming federal deficit and the danger of insolvency of the Medicare trust fund may have been the immediate impetus for this legislative speed, the chronically inflated cost of hospital treatment must be seen as the primary, longstanding problem whose time for resolution had finally come.

Thus, the rapidity of DRG's transformation from theory into law stands as an object lesson for all skeptics concerning the potential impact of ideas on social action. What remains to be seen is whether and how nursing can adapt to these sweeping changes. To do this, nursing must meet the challenge of an expanded professional identity to include the increased managerial and financial capability demanded by prospective billing.

To help achieve such an understanding of the changes that have occurred, this article will focus on the following four areas:

• A political and historical perspective on DRGs as they were applied in New Jersey, and on the prospective payment system of reimbursement.

• The research that was conducted on this system at Yale University.

• The piloting of DRG projects based on the Yale research in New Jersey and other selected states.

• The final passage of federal legislation mandating the Health Care Financing Administration's (HCFA) prospective billing for hospital care nationwide.

POLITICAL AND HISTORICAL PERSPECTIVE

Rationale for Focusing on New Jersey

The HCFA legislation arose as a response to patterns of inflation in the health care industry that reflected inflation of prices nationwide. However, in comparison to the overall economy, health care inflation has been greater. Prospective reimbursement programs designed to check this inflation in health care, however, have varied greatly from state to state. Not all programs have had the same element of prospectivity or the same organizational structures and procedural criteria for setting rates. A 1980 HCFA study, *The National Hospital Rate-Setting Study: A Comparative Review of Nine Prospective Rate-Setting Programs,* recognized this is concluding that no one generic model of rate setting guarantees a stringent, equitable program in all states. The HCFA report further noted,

> A review of the forces that prompted the adoption of prospective reimbursement programs in the nine study states reveals only one common thread: an overall concern about the escalation of hospital costs.[1]

Given this fact, a comprehensive effort to sort out the issues of prospective reimbursement on the national level creates problems in tracing the system's history through a baffling maze of regional variations. For the sake of clarity, then, we will focus on the events that took place in the State of New Jersey that led to the institution of prospective billing. Eight other states—Arizona, Connecticut, Maryland, Massachusetts, Minnesota, New York, western Pennsylvania, and Washington—also participated in the early experimentation with alternative methods of reimbursement. The New Jersey program that will be reviewed is a detailed examination of one state's experience, and is presented as an example of the complexity of nationwide prospective billing reform.

---

[1] Health Care Financing Administration. *The National Hospital Rate-Setting Study: A Comparative Review of Nine Prospective Rate-Setting Programs* (Washington, DC: Health Care Financing Administration Office of Research, Demonstrations, and Statistics, 1980).

Hill-Burton and the Post-World War II Boom

While hospitals have been accused of being the major source of national health care price escalation, a closer look reveals an historical trend toward uncontrolled budgetary expansion tracing back to the 1940s.

The federal Hill-Burton program, which had been enacted in 1946, provided the impetus for a massive postwar replenishment of hospital capital facilities.[2] Utilization of these facilities was ensured and encouraged by the Medicare and Medicaid legislation of the mid-1960s. The increasingly prominent role of other third party payers—Blue Cross, Blue Shield, and the major insurance companies—similarly led to disincentives for cost containment. Patients, physicians, and hospitals were aware that a third party payer, and not the patient, would be paying for most of the bill. This was the mood set in the days when no one envisioned sky-rocketing medical costs.

At present, hospital costs continue to rise rapidly at rates higher than the general inflation. In 1983, hospital costs increased 12.6 percent, while the general economy rate of inflation dropped to 3.9 percent. When third party payments replaced personal health care expenditures as the predominant means of paying for health care, the consumer became insulated from the true cost of health care.

In addition to third party payers' encouragement of consumer demand, their method of reimbursing hospitals was also responsible for skyrocketing costs. Because there were no effective limits on the costs to be reimbursed, the hospital was essentially guaranteed payment without having to worry about cost containment. The third party insurers and government agencies made payments to hospitals based on estimated operating costs, with retroactive adjustments allowed for each accounting period. The more a hospital spent, the more reimbursement it received from third party payers. The sky was the limit and the hospitals, run as profit-seeking institutions, took full advantage of this.

Background of New Jersey

The State of New Jersey has long upheld a tradition of legislation geared to the regulation of hospital costs in the best interests of the public.[3] This tradition goes back to 1938 when the state legislature enacted laws requiring the regulation of payment rates to assure the reasonableness and adequacy of hospital charges to major carriers. When costs began to climb in the early 1960s, the State Commissioner of Banking and Insurance responded by establishing maximum per diem rates for hospitals throughout the state. This, however, was ineffectual; hospitals arbitrarily determined what they would charge— and continued to elevate their rates at their own pace.

---

[2] R. Ullman and G. F. Kominski, "Hospital Reimbusement in the State of New Jersey." Unpublished case study, New York: Sloan Foundation, 1981.

[3] R. Caterinicchio and J. Warren, "DRGs and Medical Practice: Meeting the Challenge of Incentive Reimbursement," *The Journal of the Medical Society of New Jersey*, 1982, pp. 895-98.

In 1967, an industry analysis showed that the 10 percent annual increases in hospital rates far exceeded hospital expenditure on patient care or capital improvement. The money was going into institutional profits. The industry's internal constraints were proving to be ineffectual.

By 1968, the New Jersey Hospital Association had succeeded in establishing an Advisory Committee to the Commissioner of Banking and Insurance. However, neither state government nor consumer representation was on this committee, with the result that the efforts of this committee established hardship rate increases retroactive to 1963.

During this time, the New Jersey Hospital Association staffed the Health Research and Educational Trust, which was a volunteer organization that functioned in a "watch-dog capacity to review hospital budgets."[4] This system, however, was criticized for lack of objectivity and yielded to legislation enabling the Departments of Health and Insurance to introduce another cost control approach (reviewed immediately below). By the end of 1969, Blue Cross had petitioned the Commissioner of Banking and Insurance for a 73 percent increase in its premiums. The climate was set for a stronger voice by state government and third party payers. This led to the research and ultimate publication of the Wharton Report.

The Wharton Report

The Wharton Report was published by the Special Council to the Commissioner of Insurance of New Jersey in 1969. Along with the enactment of the Health Facilities Planning Act and the establishment of the Health Care Administration Board in 1971, this report marked the turning point in the history of New Jersey hospital rate setting. The report recommended three reforms:

1. Full prospective rate setting,
2. More direct public and consumer input to policymaking, and
3. The use of per case reimbursement methods as an alternative to the per diem method.[5]

The most important effect of the Wharton Report was to stimulate policymakers toward what was to become case-mix-based reimbursement.

Prospective Rate Setting

It is important to understand the components of prospective, as opposed to retrospective, rate setting. Dowling notes that, under a prospective rate-setting system, "providers are paid at rates set in advance of and considered fixed

---

[4] P. G. Morrison and R. P. Caterinicchio, "Case Mix Project," *New Jersey Nurse,* September/October 1980, pp. 1, 7, 10.

[5] Caterinicchio and Warren, *op. cit.*

for the pertinent period (typically a year.)"[6] Some external authority (such as the State of New Jersey) must be empowered to supervise rate setting. Dowling summarizes the concept in four steps:

1. An external authority is empowered (by statute, market power, or voluntary compliance by providers) to set provider charges and/or third party payment rates.

2. Rates are set in advance of the prospective year during which they apply and are considered fixed for the year (except for major, uncontrollable occurrences).

3. Patients and/or third parties pay the prospective rates rather than the costs actually incurred by providers during the year (or charges adjusted to cover these costs).

4. Providers are at risk for losses or surpluses.[7]

In short, prospective rates are a means of exerting more external influence over hospital activities and plans and a means of building cost containment contraints and/or incentives into hospital payment.

The Health Facilities Planning Act

The Health Facilities Planning Act of 1971 gave the Commissioner of Health great latitude to protect the consumer from unreasonable hospital charges and unreasonable hospital accounting practices. Of course, what was reasonable or unreasonable could largely depend upon who happened to be in office at the time—the Planning Act achieved scant implementation through the early part of 1974. Nonetheless, the Commissioner of Health and the Commissioner of Insurance were empowered to regulate Blue Cross charges.

Bureaucratic Malpractice

In 1974, a consumer research center published a report entitled *Bureaucratic Malpractice,* which attacked the state as being timid in exercising cost-containment efforts.[8] The report cited the per diem method of hospital reimbursement by third party payers—Blue Cross/Blue Shield, Medicare, and Medicaid—as having created an incentive for hospitals to extend the lengths of inpatient stays beyond the point of justifiable medical need. Indeed, the hospitals had every incentive to do this. They were being evaluated by insurers as businesses; the longer they could encourage patients to stay, the higher their

---

[6] W. L. Dowling, "Prospective Rate Setting: Concept and Practice," *Topics in Health Care Financing,* 3(2):8, 1979.

[7] *Ibid.*

[8] P. Powell, "Fee-for-Service," *Nursing Management,* 14(3):13-9, 1983.

profits, and the more willing third party payers were to extend themselves to pay. Blue Cross/Blue Shield, Medicare, and Medicaid all continued to raise their rates, and consumers suffered the burden of the increase.

The report suggested that reimbursement to hospitals by the "case" rather than by the day would lead to greater efficiency. This theme, formerly heard as a whisper, continued to echo louder and louder in the legislative and executive halls of New Jersey government as health care costs soared. The election of Brendan Byrne as governor in 1974 and his appointment of Joanne Finley as Health Commissioner ensured this more aggressive approach to cost containment, as recommended in the Wharton Report.

Finley and SHARE: The Last Attempt at Regulation by Per Diem

The 1970s saw a trend toward institutional change not only in hospitals, but also in other established bureaucracies that were forced into transition by practical necessity. While Joanne Finley entered office committed to controlling health care costs, her strategy for approaching this challenge altered during her tenure. Her first approach, SHARE, reviewed below, employed the traditional per diem method of billing *regulation*. This, like the preceding series of regulatory measures outlined above, operated within a system that was designed to discourage cost reduction incentives. It was found, essentially by trial and error, that only by *reform*—in this case in the implementation of DRGs—could cost escalation be reduced.

Finley's first step was to introduce public accounting into hospital reimbursement. This involved a uniform hospital accounting system imposed by the state called Standard Hospital Accounting and Rate Evaluation (SHARE).

Under the SHARE system, costs were grouped into 34 cost centers according to uniform definitions of functional centers, such as laboratory and radiology. Inpatient costs were then regrouped into 3 basic categories: 1) non-physician-controllable costs; 2) physician costs (for example, physician and resident salaries and fees); and 3) other costs that were either not controllable by the hospital or which were not to be included in the determination of the SHARE reimbursement rate. Salary rates were "equalized" in order to avoid distortions incurred by geographic wage differentials, and controllable costs were assigned to three cost-center clusters to allow for trade-offs in treatment modes. Hospital peer groups were formed and cost screens were set for each cluster of cost centers in each peer group.

After a hospital's reasonable costs were determined, a preliminary per diem reimbursement rate was determined for the hospital. This proposed SHARE per diem was reexamined in an informal review, often followed by appeals to the Department of Health and even the courts. The essential feature here was "peer grouping." This technique was developed in the utilities field. Similar institutions were classified according to their comparable attributes in order to apply "fair" standards.

Hospitals, however, are more complex than power plants and telephone companies and lend themselves less readily to accurate assessment by this method. Peer grouping may work when the basis of reimbursement is metered electricity or telephone time consumed, but hospital days render output measurable by so many indices as to confound peer review purely on the basis of one-day units of expenditure. How can a group of hospital personnel, all looking to protect their profits for every incentive imaginable, realistically be expected to accurately assign a dollar value to an imaginary hospital day? These people will operate to cover all possible costs, not to reduce them. That the activity conducted during that "day" somehow had to be worked into the equation if costs were to be controlled increasingly became apparent to New Jersey regulators.

The Yale Study. As research team members Fetter, Skin, Freeman, Averill, and Thompson note in the original DRG proposal written at Yale—the one on which many of characteristics of the HCFA system are modeled—

> The fundamental problem in cost containment is defining the appropriate tools for measuring reasonable efficiency and effectiveness in the hospital setting. Accurate instruments are needed to measure the level of productivity and effectiveness in terms both of outputs (specific services provided in terms of hours of nursing care, medications, and laboratory tests) and inputs (labor, material, and equipment used in the provision of these services) and to respond with the appropriate financial incentives or disincentives. *The attempt to measure and compare hospital efficiency at the cost-center level fails to recognize the role of case mix in determining hospital costs. Differences or lack of differences in hospital costs at the cost-center (e.g., laboratory or x-ray services) can be the result of different case mix compositions and may not reflect differences in hospital productivity* [emphasis added].[9]

These researchers also note that per diem billing tends to encourage longer lengths of stay. Emphasizing the importance of measuring and balancing the placement of incentives in the system to encourage saving rather than waste, they state,

> The reasonable measure of a hospital financial manager's effectiveness is his success in maximizing reimbursement. The more cost is increased, the greater the revenues. Costs can be skillfully redistributed over different cost centers with the effect of escaping peer cost screens. Another problem for the regulator, and opportunity for the ambitious financial manager, results from a system in which some patients pay costs (for nursing care) and others pay charges (for medical care), compounded because the ratio of costs to charges can be manipulated. Some opportunities for business gamesmanship will doubtless be found in any reimbursement methodology. The reimbursement system must identify appropriate costs and design a financial incentive to monitor and minimize such practices.[10]

Under SHARE, communications between hospital financial systems and physi-

---

[9] R. B. Fetter, Y. Shin, J. Freeman, R. Averill, and J. Thompson, "Case Mix Definition by Diagnois-Related Groups," *Medical Care,* 18(2):1-53, 1980.

[10] *Ibid.,* p. 34.

cians were discouraged principally because the plan split hospital cost information into two categories: costs directly related to patient care, and institutional and other costs. It is interesting that nursing, managerial services, facilities maintenance, and allied health costs were grouped together as institution costs.

The rationale for abandoning SHARE's per diem methodology became increasingly clear. While SHARE was a step toward cost containment and an innovative model of prospective reimbursement, it failed to introduce sufficiently powerful cost containment encouragement. The New Jersey Hospital Association actively opposed any further imposition of controls upon rates—because profits depended upon per diem billing to cover costs.

Thus, the stage was set for the introduction of DRG prospective case-mix billing into New Jersey health care. It must be seen that the most significant development in the history of hospital billing in New Jersey was the conceptual dichotomy between per diem and diagnosis related billing. Clarifying how this dichotomy developed and understanding its practical importance has been the purpose of this section.

Efforts to contain cost escalation arising from a reimbursement system that ignored the complexity of billable variables that comprise a "day" finally resulted in the conceptual leap to *reform* and to abandon *regulation*. The institutional inertia and bureaucratic resistance to this reform had resulted in a systemic preference for *covering* costs rather than *reducing* costs.

The Rise of Case Mix and the Diagnosis Related Group as Solutions to High Cost Billing: The Yale Study

The concept of staging a disease to develop homogeneous patient groups was first conceived by John Fothergill as early as 1748.[11] More recently the conceptual leap to explicitly defining the stage or the diagnosis of illness as a means of defining case mix has been developed by many different researchers.[12-18]

---

[11] M. Plomann, *Nine Patient Classification Schemes: Development, Description, and Testing* (Chicago: Health Research and Educational Trust, 1982).

[12] J. D. Bentley and P. Butler, "Measurement of Case Mix," *Topics in Health Care Financing,* 8(4):1-12, 1982.

[13] R. G. Evans, "Behavioral Cost Functions for Hospitals," *Canadian Journal of Economics,* 4(2):198-215, 1971.

[14] M. S. Feldstein, "Hospital Cost Variations and Case Mix Differences," *Medical Care,* 3(2):95-103, 1965.

[15] J. S. Gonnella, D. Z. Louis, and J. J. McCord, "The Staging Concept—An Approach to the Assessment of Outcome of Ambulatory Care, *Medical Care,* 14(1):13-21, 1976.

[16] L. D. Goodisman, and T. Trompeter, "Hospital Case Mix and Average Charge Per Case: An Initial Study," *Health Services Research,* 14(1):44-55, 1979.

[17] J. R. Lave, and L. B. Lave, "The Extent of Role Differentiation Among Hospitals," *Health Services Research,* 6:15-38, 1971.

[18] J. R. Lave, and S. Leinhardt, "The Cost and Length of a Hospital Stay," *Inquiry,* 13:327-343, 1976.

Case mix by disease staging and case mix by diagnosis are two distinct concepts, as Bentley and Butler note,

> Unlike DRGs, which rely on statistical measures (primarily based on length of stay) for grouping diagnoses, disease stages are based on physician judgments of the progression of a condition through levels of severity.[19]

Prior to 1965, researchers examining hospital case mix were primarily interested in the types of questions that per diem billing raised: What is the hospital's bed size? What is the average patient length of stay? Is the hospital a teaching hospital? The work conducted by Feldstein changed this emphasis. First demonstrating the significance of case mix in explaining variations in hospital cost, he specified the following criteria as necessary for case-mix management:

1. Patient categories must be meaningful medically, not merely convenient administratively.

2. Patient categories must be homogeneous with respect to the resources that are consumed in treatment.[20]

Feldstein argued that diagnostic categories would form a medical basis for patient grouping that was more suitable than ward assignment. Resource consumption measurement was shifted by Feldstein's research to the patient diagnostic stage, or episode, rather than the patient day.

In New Jersey, Joanne Finley was at the brink of departure from SHARE, the state's last full-blown per diem billing system. According to Grimaldi, the newly mandated approach ushered in by the passage of New Jersey Public Law 1978, Chapter 83, differed from SHARE in several important respects:

> First, the SHARE per diem method has been replaced by payment rates that depend upon the cost of treating specific cases or patients; these case-mix rates are the same regardless of the length of time most patients are hospitalized. Second, whereas SHARE sets payment rates for inpatient services received by Blue Cross and Medicaid patients, the new approach applies to all payers and all outpatient services. In short, the State now has control over all charges for inpatient and outpatient care. This control is expected to reduce cross-subsidization between payers and across services. Under SHARE, hospitals usually charge higher prices to patients for whom rates were not set, especially when Medicaid and other payers paid less than full cost. The new method requires all payers to pay essentially the same price for the same services.[21]

Thus, the state finally succeeded in eliminating much of the financial gamesmanship that SHARE allowed in inflating costs. All rates, including the

---

[19] J. Bentley and P. Butler, "Case Mix Reimbursement: Measures, Applications, Experiments," *Hospital Financial Management*, 3:14, 1980.

[20] Feldstein, *op. cit.*, p. 95.

[21] P. Grimaldi, "Equity and Efficiency Implications of Case Mix Reimbursements in New Jersey," in G. L. Glandon and R. J. Shapiro (eds.), *Profiles of Medical Practice, 1980* (Chicago: American Medical Association, Center for Health Services Research and Development, 1980), p. 93.

previously lucrative Blue Cross and Medicaid rates, were restricted by the State. Joanne Finley had emerged victorious in a lengthy political battle. It remained to be seen how the DRG system would operate to curtail the price spiral that had occurred under the per diem method. While the number of days that a patient stayed in the hospital remained at the heart of the DRG rate-setting methodology, the averaged cost of such treatment was assigned to purportedly homogeneous diagnostic categories.

The Yale Study and the Importance of Length of Stay

The developers of DRG recognized that length of stay (LOS) "may not be as accurate an indicator of the level of output as actual costs."[22] These researchers justified using it, however, because of its practical availability. Actual costs are considered to be the ideal measure of output. If, for example, a nurse paid $22,000 annually works with a patient for fifteen minutes using equipment worth X dollars, and administering X drugs, an ideal accounting system could account precisely for the dollar amount assigned to such treatment.

These data, however, for use with DRGs, do not yet exist. With the need for the practical implementation of the program as urgent as it was, length of stay was substituted by the Yale research team as the principle determinant of the cost of treating statistically determined diagnostic categories. This underscores the reason that DRGs were selected by Joanne Finley as the case-mix measure for implementation in New Jersey. As the Hospital Research and Educational Trust Working Paper Number 5 notes,

> Case mix . . . has become a misunderstood and misused concept. For many health care managers the term is synonymous with Diagnosis Related Groups (DRGs), the most popular of several patient classification systems. For others, it represents a method of hospital reimbursement by third party payers. Case mix is neither. It is a way of defining a hospital's "product" or output by identifying clinically homogeneous groups of patients that utilize similar "bundles" of treatments, tests, and services. Case-mix is a methodology that is administratively useful for partitioning patient services and determining resource allocation.[23]

Applications of case mix, presumably in relation to its confusion with DRG, troubled these researchers, who were preoccupied with the broad conceptualization of a management information system. It must be understood, however, that in the state of New Jersey, the DRG research conducted by Fetter *et al.* provided the major and immediate impetus for the transition from per diem to case-mix billing. And to return to the previously raised point, the reason that the DRG version of case-mix was selected over other case-mix alternatives reviewed by two studies in particular (Bentley and Butler, 1980; Plomann 1980), is that it confronted the practical necessity of employing length of stay as the

[22] Ullman and Kominski, *op. cit.,* p. 16.

[23] Hospital Research and Educational Trust. Working paper number 5. "The Case for Case-Mix: A New Construct for Hospital Management," September 11, 1981, p. 22.

indicator of cost for the statistical creation of the diagnostic categories. Fetter did, however, qualify their choice, acknowledging the theoretical inferiority of LOS to actual cost data: "If cost information is readily available and well standardized, that would be a preferable alternative to length-of-stay as the output utilization measure."[24] These cost data, made increasingly available with the proliferation of computer technology, may serve as the basis for a reformulation of the DRGs in the future. Nobody, however, seems to have raised the possibility of postponing implementation until these data become available when DRGs could be based upon cost; the need for containment in New Jersey, as in the rest of the country, has been too pressing.

CONCEPTUALIZING DRG: CATEGORIES AND STRATEGIES

The DRG system has been approached by the health care professionals with a sense of mystery that the complexity of its origin has generated. This section will outline the goals of DRG, its principal categories, and the strategies for their implementation.

The hospital product. First, and most important, DRG is an attempt to define a "product" of an industry that had previously neglected to do so. This product is comprised of the specific set of outputs received by patients. The "output" that the hospital provides is defined in such terms as hours of nursing care, medications, laboratory tests, and so forth. The costs, or "inputs," required for the creation or provision of this service-output are labor (including nursing and other staff salaries) and materials and equipment used.[25]

Different patients receive different amounts and types of services that heretofore were priced inaccurately under the per diem system of reimbursement. By conceptualizing the hospital output as "products" used by different patients, the authors of the DRG proposal conceptualize the hospital as a multiproduct firm, "with a product line that in theory is as extensive as the number of patients it serves."[26] The particular product purchased, selected, or provided is defined by the researchers in terms of diagnosis. Some "products" require more hospital resources than others and are therefore considered to be more complex—and expensive. The relative proportions of the various types of cases treated by a particular hospital are called its case mix.

Internal management of efficiency and effectiveness are not served by the per diem criteria of hospital performance, which have been aggregate indicators: cost per patient day, percent occupancy, and mortality rate. Patient days of care and number of admissions or discharges have been used to describe hospital output under the per diem system. (Table 1 compares the two methods of measuring hospital product.)

According to Fetter, diagnosis related groups were developed "to evaluate, compare, and provide relevant feedback regarding hospital performance."[27]

---

[24] Fetter *et al.*, *op. cit.*   [26] *Ibid.*, p. 1.

[25] *Ibid.*, p. 17.   [27] *Ibid.*, p. 2.

Table 1.
Comparison of Traditional and DRG Reimbursement Systems

	Traditional	DRG
Payment mechanism is:	Per diem, or total hospital costs divided by patient days	By the case, or costs related to treatment of specific DRG
Payment unit is:	The patient day	The diagnosis
Calculation of rates:	Rates reflect hospital's own costs	Rates are derived from a blending of hospital-specific amounts based on each hospital's cost experience. National and regional (for nine census divisions) DRG amounts for both urban and rural hospitals. Transitional period— by October 1, 1986, payment will be 100% of the national urban or rural DRG rate.
Time frame:	Retrospective	Prospective
System incentives:	Hospital has limited incentive to contain costs, since expenses are reimbursed retrospectively	Hospital profits from cost containment through receipt of "incentive" payments when length of stay is lower than "average" and experiences "disincentives" when costs exceed the standard.
Payers:	Commercial payers are billed for costs disallowed by noncommercial payers	The system will apply to all Medicare participating hospitals, except psychiatric, long-term care, rehabilitation, and children's hospitals, and hospitals outside the 50 states and Washington, DC.

Source: Adapted from the 1982 Annual Report of the New Jersey
Rate Setting Commission.

To do this they require identification of the specific products provided by the institution. In order to treat the large numbers of consumers demanding hospital products, the "consumers" must be classified by type. The method for defining these consumer types is classification by case diagnosis, demographic characteristics; and therapeutic attributes. The researchers note,

> The means of defining hospital case mix for this purpose is the construction and application of a classification scheme comprised of subgroups of patients possessing similar clinical attributes and output utilization patterns. This involves relating demographic, diagnostic and therapeutic characteristics of patients to the output they are provided so that cases are differentiated by only those variables related to the condition of the patient (e.g., age, primary diagnosis) and treatment process (e.g., operations) that affect his utilization of the hospital's facilities.[28]

The researchers then note, in one sentence, the major cost-saving and managerial components of the DRG system: "These groups or patient classes may then be useful for certain applications in patient care *monitoring, budgeting, cost control, reimbursement, and planning*" [emphasis added].[29] These cost control features, oriented to clinically based diagnostic categories, assign cost-accounting indexes and managerial strategies to the hospital product. For the first time, the hospital has become an industry with a product the price of which can be managed and monitored by the caregivers themselves as the product is dispensed.

The researchers determined that the classification scheme should have the following attributes:

1. It must be interpretable medically, with subclasses of patients from homogeneous diagnostic categories. That is, when the patient classes are described to physicians, they should be able to relate to these patients and be able to identify a particular patient management process for them.

2. Individual classes should be defined on variables that are commonly available in hospital abstracts and are relevant to output utilization, pertaining to either the condition of the patient or the treatment process.

3. There must be a manageable number of classes, preferably in the hundreds instead of thousands, that are mutually exclusive and exhaustive. That is, they must cover the entire range of possible disease conditions in the acute-care setting without overlap.

4. The classes should contain patients with similar expected measures of output utilization.

5. Class definitions must be comparable, with similar expected measures of output utilization.[30]

---

[28] *Ibid.*

[29] *Ibid.*

[30] *Ibid.*

The classification categories were coded using the *International Classification of Diseases, Adapted for Use in the United States, Eighth Revision (ICDAS)* and the *Hospital Adaptation of ICDA, Second Edition (HICDA2)*. These coding schemes, "provide a classification of conditions of morbidity and mortality for statistical reporting purposes as well as for information retrieval."[31]

The first version of the diagnosis related group system included 383 categories. Bentley and Butler note four advantages of this system:

1. DRGs are conceptually appealing because they attempt to describe patterns of resource consumption based on the similarities and differences among patients.

2. The classification is based upon data generally included in the discharge abstract.

3. The method results in a manageable number of diagnostic categories, which is 383.

4. DRGs are organized in an hierarchical manner. The terminal diagnostic groups can be collapsed into fewer categories that, while more heterogeneous, are still useful.[32]

Bentley and Butler also note five major disadvantages of the system:

1. DRGs rely upon discharge abstracts, which often contain classification and coding errors. Furthermore, DRGs fail to include all diagnoses and procedures. Assignment to a DRG is dependent upon the documentation of the attending physician and the conventions of the individual coder.

2. DRGs reflect the state of medical technology and practice at the time of their development; therefore, to account for advances in diagnostic procedures and treatment modalities, DRGs have to be reformulated.

3. The performance of a surgical procedure often categorizes a patient into a more complex DRG. If DRGs are used for reimbursement and if the reimbursement method reflects the complexity of the DRG, surgical procedures may be encouraged because they result in higher reimbursement.

4. DRGs only group and classify inpatients.

5. DRGs group patients into categories asserted to be homogeneous on the basis of length of stay data. Thus, DRGs are neither a standard of what should be done nor a measure of the quality of care.[33]

---

[31] *Ibid.*

[32] Bentley and Butler, *op. cit.*

[33] *Ibid.*

Problems. Researchers have continued to find problems with the DRGs. Some have attacked the categories for lacking homogeneity. Others attack the lack of applicability of LOS (length of stay) to actual cost. Some applicants for reimbursement found that the categories were applicable only among the population originally tested. Others found that the age categories were not sharply enough defined. Because of these problems and others, in 1979 Yale researchers reformulated the DRGs using a new coding scheme *(International Classification of Diseases-9-CM).*

Efforts toward solutions. As a result, a new categorization of diseases was produced that attempted to alleviate the problems. A national data base was employed to accommodate the regional objections to DRG applications. The Major Diagnostic Categories (MDCs) were reduced from 83 to 23. This change attempted to describe more closely the organization of medical practice according to medical specialty. Accommodation was made for outliers—that is, cases that do not fall into DRGs. Surgery was reclassified by presence in operating room and its categories were refined in the endeavor to reduce fraudulent upgrading of other diagnoses to merit surgery's higher reimbursement rates. Age was used more consistently.

After revision, the Yale researchers listed some of their assessments of the DRG weaknesses, and this produced a picture of an imperfect system painted by its own creators. Some homogeneity, in terms of discreteness, was admitted to be sacrificed for the sake of maintaining a manageable number of groups. Some of the dependence upon physician opinion to accommodate the classification scheme's goal of matching medical categories produced vulnerability to differences in therapeutic philosophy. Physicians may vary in their treatment of the same disease, and different treatment methods have different costs. Some diseases have no common treatment regimes. Some of the discharge abstracts lack staging of the disease. Readmission proves difficult when this information is absent. The population size of some small hospitals makes some categories meaningless.

Outliers and trim points. One of the reasons that the original 383 categories were redefined was that there were excessive numbers of "outliers" or patients who did not fit into any category. Joel notes that "trim points," or designated variance for each DRG, mark the bounds of allocation of the DRG's dollar amount.[34] If a diagnosis requires more or less expenditure than such an amount, the patient reverts to the traditional per diem and charge model. If the patient is discharged under the variance because of recovery, death, or interagency transfer, the full rate is not charged. Patients staying beyond the outer limits of the DRG are billed on a per diem basis. These outliers must be certified. This is to prevent the system's reversion to a completely per diem orientation by unanimous application for outlier status.

Connor raises the excellent point that with all New Jersey hospitals com-

---

[34] L. Joel, "Case Mix Reimbursement: DRGs, RIMs," *The Massachusetts Nurse,* January 1983, pp. 5-6.

peting to maximize profits by charging less than the DRG state averages (and still getting paid the DRG amount), the state average may well decline as a result. If the average declines, will competition really increase the hospitals' profits, or will the average only continue to descend and destroy profit dollars? Is the DRG method of reimbursement harboring long-run disincentives? Connor thus wisely recommends the intervention of a regulatory intermediary to ensure that public input determines a "floor beneath which the payment standard is not allowed to fall."[35]

Effect on Nursing

Several case-mix demonstration projects have included a nursing component, one of the most recent being the Case-Mix Nursing Performance Study executed during 1979 and 1980, and reviewed further below. The outcomes of the Case-Mix Nursing Performance Study were used to generate Relative Intensity Measures (RIMs) of nursing consumption.[36]

DRG AS A MANAGEMENT INFORMATION SYSTEM

In addition to the Yale DRG study's statement of the cost-saving and managerial components of the DRG system, Bisbee and Bachofer underline the importance of the very structure of the DRG system itself as a management tool. They note,

> Case mix is important for management purposes because, along with the volume of patients admitted during the year, it influences the resources that a hospital will use. Staffing levels, capital equipment, and the type and quantity of supplies to be ordered are all influenced by the type of patients that will be admitted to the hospital. An effective case-mix system could enable the administrator to analyze the types of patients being admitted, to estimate the amount and type of resources required to treat those patients, and to monitor performance based on the types of patients actually admitted.[37]

They add that there are four potential management applications of case mix information:

---

[35] R. Connor, "Case-based Payment Systems: Eight Indicators to Watch," *Hospital & Health Services Administration,* 27:43, 1982.

[36] Morrison and Caterinicchio, *op. cit.*

[37] G. Bisbee and H. Bachofer, "Usefulness of Case Mix Systems as a Tool in Hospital Management Must Be Determined," *Hospital Services Research,* 2(2):28-31, 1979.

1. Resource allocation, including planning and budgeting.
2. Pricing, including rate setting and financial planning.
3. Cost and efficiency control, including standard setting, measurement of performance, and productivity management.
4. Quality control, including utilization review and quality assurance.[38]

THE HCFA PROSPECTIVE PAYMENT PLAN

What then does the HCFA plan have to do with all of this? New Jersey's plan, in requiring fixed ceilings on reimbursements for all payers, set the stage for the HCFA model.

On or after October 1, 1983, Medicare payment for inpatient operating costs will be based on a fixed amount, determined in advance, for each case, according to one of 467 diagnosis related groups into which a case is classified. The prospective payment will be considered payment in full; hospitals are prohibited from charging beneficiaries more than the statutory deductible and coinsurance.

The HCFA Prospective Payment Policy replaces, for most hospitals, the retrospective cost-reimbursement system, the cost-per-case limits, and the rate-of-increase ceiling created by the Tax Equity and Fiscal Responsibility Act of 1982 (TEFRA), P.L. 97-248. In addition, through fiscal year 1985, payments for Medicare inpatient hospital costs under the prospective payment system will be no more or less than those projected under the TEFRA provisions.

As in New Jersey, cost data from previous years will be used by HCFA to develop a fixed rate per DRG. Medicare will pay a hospital a flat rate for each of 467 DRGs. If patient treatment in a DRG category costs a hospital less than this rate, the hospital keeps the surplus as a profit. This is the first time that the government has endorsed such profit-making by non-profit hospitals. If, however, patient treatment in a DRG category costs a hospital more than the prespecified Medicare DRG rate, the hospital absorbs the loss. Because of the varying expertise of different hospitals in various diagnostic categories, there will be DRGs that will make money for some hospitals and lose money for others.

Overall, the HCFA plan will incorporate those elements of the programs, piloted in New Jersey and other states, that can be easily administered on a national level. Discharged patients will be categorized into 467 groups based upon diagnosis, age, treatment procedure, discharge status, and sex. The program will begin nationwide on the hospitals' first accounting period on or after October 1, 1983. It will progress in a "stepped" or "layered" fashion, phasing in over a three-year period, as follows:

- In the first year, 25 percent of the payment will be based on regional DRG rates, and a 75 percent weighting will be based on the hospital's historic cost experience.

---

[38] *Ibid.*

- In the second year, 50 percent of the payment will be based on a combination of national and regional DRG rates (25 percent national, 75 percent regional); 50 percent of the payment will be based on each hospital's cost experience.

- In the third year, 75 percent of the payment will be based on a combination of national and regional DRG rates (50 percent national, 50 percent regional); 25 percent of the payment will be based on each hospital's cost experience.

- By the fourth year, 100 percent of the payment will be based upon national DRG rates.

In contrast with the New Jersey DRG prospective payment system, the national system will apply only to Medicare, not to all third-party payers. The national DRG category rates will be adjusted for rural and urban hospitals within nine census regions. Further, in addition to hospitals' historical cost data, rates will be based on annual industry-wide increases in hospital costs. For example, rates will be updated in fiscal years 1984 and 1985 using an index of the costs of goods and services purchased by hospitals plus one percentage point. After fiscal year 1985, DRG rate increases will be set according to the opinion of a commission of experts.

Also, in contrast with New Jersey's implementation, under the HCFA Prospective Payment Policy capital-related costs will be excluded from the prospective rate and will be progressively instituted as follows:

- For the first three years of implementation, capital costs other than return on equity will be reimbursed on a reasonable basis.

- Return on equity will be reimbursed at the same rate as the average interest rate on the Medicare Hospital Insurance Trust Fund, which is down one-and-one-half times from the current rate.

- After October 1, 1986, all capital costs, including return on equity, will be prospectively reimbursed.

Direct and indirect teaching costs will be dealt with in a manner similar to that in New Jersey.

- Direct teaching costs—including the costs of nursing education programs—will continue to be paid on a reasonable-cost basis. They will be excluded from the prospective payment determinations.

- Indirect teaching expenses will be reimbursed at twice the amount of the teaching adjustment under the Tax Equity Fiscal Responsibility Act (TEFRA).

New Jersey has implemented an extensive appeals process by which hospitals that believe they have somehow been misclassified under one DRG category or another can appeal these decisions. The appeal process is limited to improvements in clinical management of patient care. While the HCFA plan requires hospitals to contract with professional review organizations to review the quality of care provided, the appropriateness of Medicare admissions, and the appropriateness of care to patients designated as outliers, the extensiveness of the appeals process seen in New Jersey has not been replicated by HCFA. It may well be that the administrative complexities of administering appeals processes compelled the legislators to leave their adoption to individual state discretion.

Concerning state options for bypassing the DRG system, the Secretary of Health and Human Services can permit alternative cost-control systems so long as these do not result in Medicare expenditures above those under the DRG system. The criteria for these systems would be discretionarily set by the Secretary. A waiver for such exceptions would be submitted to the Secretary.

Excerpted from the HCFA Prospective Payment Plan would be psychiatric, long-term care, and children's and rehabilitation hospitals. Also excepted would be hospitals in Puerto Rico and U.S. territories.

Physicians, as in New Jersey, will not be reimbursed according to medical diagnoses. The Secretary, however, will be required to collect data and to report to Congress concerning this issue by December 31, 1984, concerning the advisability and feasibility of including physician payments in DRG rates.

Quality control and system monitoring are to be implemented in relation to admission patterns and DRG categories. This kind of monitoring is already part of the cost limit program required by the 1982 law. For prospective payment, the medical review mechanism will identify unusual changes in the volume of admissions, case mix, total reimbursement, and discharge status. The cause of any such fluctuations will be investigated. Additionally, a system of DRG verification will be implemented to assure that the DRGs assigned to individual cases are correct, focusing in particular on their tendency to ''creep'' on into costlier classifications or ''skimming'' and only admitting the most profitable client.

The HCFA payment system will provide for a review of the prospective payment system itself by the Congressional Office of Technology Assessment (OTA). The OTA director is to appoint a 15-member commission of experts by 1984, including representation by physicians, nurses, other health professionals, hospitals, business groups, and others. The commission will advise the Congress and the Secretary on prospective payment matters.

CONCLUSION

As Bisbee stated, ''A change to DRG-based reimbursement would involve a major repositioning of the 'carrots and sticks' that influence hospital behavior.''[39] In this sense, the new system will plunge health care into the com-

---

[39] Bisbee, *op. cit.*

petitive world of business. The system's incentives for efficiency along with the decreasing demand for inpatient hospital services will be the forces driving health care toward a competitive marketplace. All of this will require health care professionals with new kinds of managerial skills. From the perspective of expenditure and percentage of the gross national product, health care is the largest business in the United States.

How nursing will adapt to the demand for professional restructuring to accommodate the requirements of this business will be considered in a future article. What is important as a beginning is that nursing professionals immediately become informed of the implications of the new legisiation that will quickly render obsolete their customary ways of looking at their work. It is true that the DRG prospective billing system will bring about a major repositioning of the "carrots and sticks" that influence hospital behavior. In New Jersey, it already has.

DRGs
AS ONE OF NINE APPROACHES
TO CASE MIX IN TRANSITION

Marilyn Peacock Plomann
Franklin A. Shaffer

The Social Security Amendments of 1983 represent a major change in the basic policies that have governed Medicare payment during the past decade. These newly established payment limitations put hospitals at risk both for the type of patient admitted for treatment and for the use of the routine and ancillary services. Under the new payment system, if a hospital's cost per case exceeds the defined limit, it will incur a loss regardless of its cost-to-charge ratio. In other words, the hospital, rather than Medicare or other third-party payer, bears the cost of longer stays and increased use of routine and ancillary services. Therefore, hospitals must look toward adopting case-based management systems to effectively manage operation.

All of this, however, is only the beginning of a series of reimbursement reforms that promise to alter the nature of medical care by the end of the century, in both degree and kind, more extensively than is currently imaginable. We are now in the midst of only the second generation of DRG case-mix reimbursement. The first generation of this prospective case-mix reimbursement system, using 383 diagnosis-related categories, was changed to the present 467 categories. The current set of DRGs is, in turn, being updated by researchers to improve the system's operation in relation to three fundamental areas: 1) hospital product definition, 2) provision of information to managers concerning the cost of resources and services, and 3) combining the administrative and financial parts of the hospital product with the clinical parts of the hospital product. Thus, the second DRG method of case-mix reimbursement is being modified as rapidly as was the first, and it can be inferred from this process that the pace is accelerating toward further improvement and streamlining of case-mix methodology.

From this standpoint, it should be noted that the DRG prospective method of case-mix reimbursement was considered by its authors to expeditiously implement quality assurance with cost control at a time when prospective reimbursement was known in only research and pilot studies.[1] The institution of the DRG method was executed rapidly as a stopgap measure to control hospital costs that had soared beyond the reach of both public and private budgetary restraint. This is particularly true in relation to length of stay, which the developers of DRG recognized as possibly not "...as accurate an indicator of the level of output as actual costs."[2] The researchers justified using it because of its practical availability at a time when costs required cutting on a near-emergency basis.

Therefore, conceptually focusing exclusively on DRGs rather than case mix as a whole would restrict forward-looking health-case managers' vision by conceptualizing as static what is proving to be a dynamic process. It would also constitute *reacting to* rather than *actively controlling* the change process itself. Understanding just where we are in case mix's developmental history, and seeing how the long history of case-mix reform is currently being interwoven with ongoing changes, requires a brief review of some of the other case mix options from which DRG was selected. Indeed, to date, nine distinct approaches using patient descriptors of case mix—diagnosis, personal characteristics, and pattern of treament—have been developed. These are:

- ICD-9-CM list A
- diagnosis related groups (DRGs)
- patient management categories
- MD-DADO
- AS-SCORE
- severity of illness index
- disease staging
- generic algorithms
- VA multilevel care groups

These approaches can be described or classified according to the purpose for which they were developed. Four objectives were behind the development of the various classification schemes: utilization review, reimbursement, quality assurance, and management applications. Because each classification system was formulated to achieve its objective, the result was nine systems that vary significantly. The information provided, or the variable explained, by each

---

[1]R.B.Y. Fetter, J. Freeman, R. Averill, and J. Thompson, "Case Mix Definition by Diagnosis-Related Groups," *Medical Care,* 8(2):12, 1980.

[2]R. Ullman and G.F. Kominski, "Hospital Reimbursement in the State of New Jersey." Unpublished case study available from Sloan Foundation. Sloan Foundation, 1981, p. 16.

system differed depending upon the system's purpose. For instance, diagnosis related groups were developed as a tool for utilization review. As mentioned above, to achieve this purpose, the developers selected length of stay as the variable to be measured. To assure widespread application, the data elements selected to explain length of stay were restricted to those captured on the patient discharge abstract.

The particular data elements used to explain the desired variable differ significantly. For example, all of the systems intended for quality assurance applications focused on measuring the severity level of disease; however, they used different data elements, or patient characteristics, to measure severity. The patient characteristics that were selected varied depending upon the philosophy and orientation of the individuals involved in developing the system.

As previously noted, there are differences among the classification systems. As a rule, each possesses strengths and weaknesses that should be considered before being applied in the hospital setting. And, as previously noted, some of the characteristics of the eight approaches that have not been adopted in the present system could well be included in future revisions of case-mix applications to what is a new way of thinking about patients, physicians, services and resource components of the hospital product. All of these are linked with financial measurement by the merging of clinical and financial data in the case mix.

ICD-9-CM LIST A

ICD-9-CM list A is based on ICD-9-CM and is an expansion of the Commission on Professional and Hospital Activities (CPHA) list A, which was based on H-ICDA-2 and which was published in 1974 by the commission. The original list A was developed to identify diagnosis groups that are useful for review and evaluation of the utilization of facilities, services, and quality of care by the hospital, the Professional Standards Review Organization, and other interested parties. The ICD-9-CM list A contains 398 diagnosis groups that are further categorized into case types or cells that are based on five age variables and dichotomies for operated/not operated and single diagnosis/multiple diagnoses. The end result is 7,960 case types of cells.

The limitation of list A that was cited most often by case-mix researchers, hospital administrators, and some utilization review agencies is that the number of case types — 7,960 — is too large, which results in many cells containing an insignificant number of patients. Other limitations not cited as often, although more important, include the equal treatment given to secondary diagnoses and the omission of specific surgical procedures. Clinically, not all secondary diagnoses will have the same effect on a patient's level of illness, but list A gives all secondary diagnoses equal weighting. List A segregates patients on the basis of operated/not operated; however, the type of surgical procedure (major versus minor) may affect a patient's use of resources. While the number of case types is unwieldy, some of the criticisms of the DRG system currently in use, reported further below, concern the different approaches that different health care managers have to finer shades and distinctions within the same diagnostic categories. When the next version of case-mix classifications emerges, it may well have drawn upon some of the 7,960 types set forth in the ICD-9-CM list A.

DIAGNOSIS RELATED GROUPS

Diagnosis related groups (DRGs) were initially developed in the late 1960s and mid-1970s at the Yale University Center for Health Studies and at Yale-New Haven Hospital. The researchers were interested in defining expected lengths of patient stays for quality-of-care studies and utilization review activities. The primary objective in the construction of DRGs was a definition of case types, each of which could be expected to receive similar amounts of services from a hospital. Length of stay was used a measure of hospital services.

In late 1981, new DRGs were developed by the Health Systems Management Group of the Yale University School of Organization and Management, under a grant from the Health Care Financing Administration. Because the 383 DRGs have been available for several years and have been used in a variety of applications, a number of advantages and disadvantages have been noted. The cited advantages include:

- DRGs are conceptually appealing because they attempt to describe patterns of resource consumption based on similarities and differences among patients.

- The classification is based on data generally included in the discharge abstract.

- The method results in a manageable number of diagnostic categories, which is 383.

- DGRs are organized in a hierarchical manner. The terminal diagnostic groups can be collapsed into fewer categories that, while more heterogeneous, are still useful.

In addition, persons who have used DRGs for internal hospital management have been able to demonstrate that changes in hospital costs can be divided into the increased cost associated with a more complex case mix and increased prices for treating the same case mix.

The major disadvantages include:

- DRGs rely on discharge abstracts, which often contain classification and coding errors. Furthermore, DRGs fail to include all diagnoses and procedures. Assignment to a DRG depends on the documentation of the attending physician and the conventions of the individual coder.

- DRGs reflect the state of medical technology and practice at the time of their development; therefore, to account for advances in diagnostic procedures and treatment modalities, DRGs will have to be reformulated.

- The performance of a surgical procedure often categories a patient into a more complex DRG. If DRGs are used for reimbursement, and if the reinbursement method reflects the complexity of the DRG, surgical procedures may be encouraged because they result in higher reimbursement.

- DRGs only group and classify inpatients.

- DRGs group patients into categories that are asserted to be homogeneous on the basis of length-of-stay data. Thus, DRGs are neither a standard of what should be done nor a measure of the quality of care.

As a result of several reimbursement applications, a number of controversies surrounding DRGs have been identified. The DRG developers have asserted that the terminal DRGs group patients who are logically similar from a broad medical viewpoint, while some users argue that DRGs are not clinically meaningful because they group together unrelated patients. For example, DRG 39 groups together all patients whose primary diagnosis is cancer of the bone, thyroid, connective tissue, and nervous system who did not receive a surgical procedure.

In addition, those who have used DRGs assert that they are not clinically meaningful because they fail to subdivide some broad diagnostic groups. For example, DRG 121 includes all patients whose primary diagnosis is acute myocardial infarction.

Another way in which DRGs have been cited as not clinically meaningful is their failure to differentiate patients in various stages of the same illness. For example, the DRGs group together, in a single category, lung cancer patients with a short diagnostic workup and those with a terminal condition.

Although DRG developers have asserted that the terminal DRGs group together patients who use similar amounts of resources, some users of DRGs argue that length of stay is not an appropriate measure of resource consumption. This was mentioned above and is reiterated here. Length of stay is correlated with price per day ($r = -.672$); however, there is little relationship between price per day and price per case. Users of DRGs also argue that the classification system fails to recognize the standby capacity needed for high-risk patients. For example, if a high-risk pregnancy results in a normal delivery, the patient is classified as a normal delivery with no recognition of the special services required to be present in the event that the risk had materialized.

Other researchers have found that DRGs are not externally valid (that is, they cannot be applied to populations other than those from which they were originally derived). Blue Cross of Western Pennsylvania applied the same statistical method used by Yale researchers to a sample of 690,000 patient records and did not produce identical terminal DRGs. The Pennsylvania researchers found that DRGs were not homogeneous because a substantial variance reduction could be achieved by further partitioning diagnostic categories. These diagnostic categories could be subdivided based on the same defining independent variable and additional variables that were not available in the original data set, such as admission class or hospital characteristics. The analysis demonstrates that heterogeneity within a DRG could not be assumed to represent differential treatment of similar patients.

Although the independent variables that were used to subdivide the major diagnostic categories into terminal DRGs included patient age, many of those using DRGs have found that patient age needed to receive greater emphasis in formulating diagnostic groups. In one major Maryland teaching hospital, Medicare patients generally consume 15 percent more resources than non-Medicare patients for the same DRG. In New York City, one teaching hospital found that its over-65 patients stayed approximately 50 percent longer than its under-65 patients in the same DRG.

Those who have attempted to use DRGs for internal management of the hospital's clinical activities have found that some DRGs often have fewer than five cases for a given year. It is difficult to make comparative or evaluative judgments with such small numbers. At one hospital with approximately 16,000 admissions in 1977, only 20 of the terminal DRGs had at least 30 cases.

The 467 new DRGs have not been tested but will be used to implement prospective payment legislation. Yale researchers have identified some difficulties in the derivation of the new DRGs:

- In an attempt to derive a manageable number of patient classes, some clinical homogeneity within groups was lost. Practicing physicians want specificity, rather than a "manageable" number of groups, because they believe that the ability to generalize decreases as the number of groups is decreased. However, a system with a large number of classes would not be administratively useful, and the marginal contribution of added classes is doubtful.

- Some of the classifying variables used to derive the terminal DRGs are medical practice variables (for example, absence or presence of cardiac catheterization during hospitalization for surgery). Therefore, DRGs may be limited from a clinical perspective because of:

    Differences in therapeutic philosophy. Physicians may vary in their treatment of the same disease, causing similar patients to use different resources in the treatment regimen.

    The absence of common treatment regimens. In the treatment of disease states, there are some with no accepted treatment regimens; therefore, the use of resources will vary.

    Lack of staging and readmission data. For utilization review and quality assurance programs, physicians would prefer data on the stage of the disease and whether the patient is a readmission. These data are not included in standard discharge data sets.

- Small hospitals may not be able to use DRGs because they may not have enough patients in some categories to make DRG data meaningful. In addition, differences in the availability of resources between small and large institutions will affect treatment patterns and perhaps length of stay. Because DRGs are based on length of stay, they may not be valid for small hospitals.

DISEASE STAGING

The concept of staging a disease to develop homogeneous patient groups was first conceived by John Fothergill in 1748. Years later, the staging concept was developed and applied in the area of cancer by the National Institute of Health (NIH). NIH realized the necessity of including the dimension of severity of illness in defining homogeneous patient clusters that could be used in clinical trials designed to test the efficacy of various cancer treatments. This concept of explicitly defining the stage of an illness is the basis for the disease-staging approach used to determine case mix, which was developed by Joseph Gonnella, MD, associate dean of Jefferson Medical College, in conjunction with SysteMetrics, Inc., of California.

Disease staging was initially designed as a tool to monitor quality of patient care by classifying patients with similar conditions and assessing their patterns of resource utilization. This method of classifying patients was developed in response to a lack of effective techniques by which to evaluate patient care. A basic deficiency of existing methods has been their inability to classify patients with similar conditions into homogeneous clusters for use in comparing physician performance and alternative methods of health care delivery. Traditionally, medical taxonomy has been based more on pathophysiological and anatomical findings than on identification of medically homogeneous patient groupings that would be useful for predicting the results of medical treatment. Disease staging attempts to add greater precision to traditional disgnostic classifications by describing, in quantitative and clinical terms, the progression of a disease or problem in terms of increasing severity.

One disadvantage in disease staging is that it does not attempt to capture all of the variables that contribute to hospital costs or resource requirements. Patient-related variables (such as age, family support, or overall health status), provider-related variables (such as choice of treatment modality and institutional capabilities), and community characteristics not captured by the staging method can have a significant impact on hospital costs. These patient-related, provider-related, and community-related variables can, and do, vary among hospitals. Disease staging, however, does attempt to isolate the major variable that determines the need for hospital resources (that is, the severity of the medical problem). By isolating this major variable, hospital managers can identify and analyze the effect of the other related variables on the utilization of resources. Once the variables that contribute to variances in resource use have been identified, managers can plan and monitor hospital resources more effectively. It is important to note that current complaints concerning the DRGs currently in use is their lack of sensitivity to the staging and progression of each diagnosis. Refinements to these groups, which will produce a new case-mix system, may well include some of the components of disease staging.

PATIENT MANAGEMENT CATEGORIES

The patient management category (PMC) approach to case mix measurement, currently in its fourth year of development, is under the direction of Wanda Young, ScD, of Blue Cross of Western Pennsylvania. PMCs are defined in terms of the reason for hospital admission and the discharge diagnosis. Patient categories are based entirely on clinical input obtained through physician consultation and panel review, as opposed to statistically derived patient categories based on length-of-stay or hospital-charge data.

Development of the PMC system is expected to be completed shortly. PMC is being tested in six hospitals, where data are being collected to aid in system evaluation. This system seems to involve physician input at the outset rather than imposing predetermined categories upon all health care managers before patients are admitted. DRGs have evolved as a more externally rigid imposition upon the system employing length of stay as their measurement basis for disease-treatment financing.

The Patient Management Categories system is based more on physician involvement, rather than on purely statistical measurements.

VA MULTI-LEVEL CARE GROUPS

Developed in 1976, although not currently in use, the Veterans Administration Department of Medicine and Surgery multilevel care system (MLC) is a refinement of the progressive patient care concept that many hospitals in the United States and Europe adopted in the late 1950s. The principal function of the MLC system is to match patients' variable health resource needs with different amounts or clusters of resources (levels of care). Health care managers can identify the average resources consumed by patients at each level of care and then determine the real costs of these resources. The MLC system was tailored to meet the needs of VA administrative and clinical managers for a reliable, yet practical, management tool that could be implemented with relative ease to allocate federal dollars among VA medical centers.

The MLC system is a useful mechanism for hospitals that have not determined costs or prices for their different products by patient. However, in hospitals where charges can be aggregated by patient, the use of only four categories, based on four hospital levels of care for the medical-surgical setting, would not provide hospitals with any additional information. In these instances, the MLC patient classification system would only be useful as a comprehensive nursing classification system because much emphasis has been given to determining the nursing component of care at each level.

By using only four categories, patients within a category are not medically homogeneous (that is, patients within one category do not evoke a set of the clinical responses that result in similar amounts and kinds of resource use). The MLC system captures the intensity or amount of resource use within a level of care; however, the type of resources will vary within the group because patients at a given level are admitted for different reasons. Two elements are important to note in this approach to case-mix management. First, this method employs relative intensity of resource use rather than length of stay as the means of determining case mix. Future case-mix systems may well look to this kind of computation of resource utilization, the accuracy of which supercedes that of length of stay for any given diagnosis. Second, the emphasis on cost allocation for nursing care is also advantageous in this approach. Currently, most DRG systems consider nursing to be part of hospital overhead and do not evaluate diagnoses according to their intensity requirements for nursing services.

AS-SCORE

The AS-SCORE classification system was developed by George Roveti, MD, and Sharon Kreitzer, RN, at Church Hospital, Baltimore, with the assistance of Susan D. Horn, PhD, of the Johns Hopkins Center for Hospital Finance and Management. AS-SCORE was developed as a tool to evaluate the appropriateness of hospital length of stay and to measure physician performance. The method classifies patients into four levels of severity, based on clinical data documented in the patient medical record at the time of discharge. AS-SCORE can be used either alone or in conjunction with other case-mix grouping methods to establish categories within disease states to account for variations caused by severity of illness.

This approach, like the Patient Management Categories system, has a certain degree of physician involvement. Any future case-mix applications must take severity of illness into account. Staging is one attempt to accomplish this end.

SEVERITY OF ILLINESS INDEX

The severity of illness index is a refinement of the AS-SCORE classification system. The refinement of AS-SCORE was undertaken to develop a severity index that is applicable to almost all hospitalized patients and that uses classifying variables that are more precisely defined and, therefore, more teachable and more reliable.

Although the severity of illness index has demonstrated its usefulness in many areas of hospital of hospital management, its major limitation is that it relies on the judgment of the individual who collects the severity data and assigns an overall severity rating to individual cases. However, researchers are investigating computerization of the severity of illness index based on an expanded discharge abstract data base.

The severity of illness index produces patient groups that are homogeneous with respect to researchers' definition of severity or burden of illness. Severity is defined and measured using seven patient attributes. These attributes have been shown to reflect resource use (that is, total charges, length of stay, laboratory charges, and routine charges). Two of these attributes (nonoperating room procedures and nursing requirements) are related to resource use but may be influenced by the hospital staff. However, researchers contend that these variables are least influential in producing the overall severity level and were included because they often reflect the burden of illness.

Like other case-mix grouping methods in use today, the severity of illness index is a retrospective rather than a prospective classification system. Patient categories are based on what occurred during hospitalization rather than on variables that are predictors of required resources.

MD-DADO

The physician discharge abstract data optimal (MD-DADO) system was developed at the Johns Hopkins Center for Hospital Finance and Management and the Rockburn Institute in Maryland. Development of the MD-DADO system was undertaken in response to a grant from the Health Care Financing Administration to explore research methods of case-mix groupings. The MD-DADO system is the result of an attempt to refine the 383 diagnosis related groups with charge per case as the dependent variable and with systematic physician input.

The MD-DADO groups represent an approach to analyzing hospital admissions rather than a universal, fixed classification system. The methodology employed allows for adjustment of the groups to reflect local factors, such as physician preferences and types of diseases characteristic of a specific patient population. The groups can therefore be adjusted to reflect the unique features of an institution. This approach involves refinement of many of the problems plaguing the current DRG system; the substitution of systematic physician input for the imposition of a fixed classification system recognized the objections that the users of the current system have raised concerning DRG applications among varying health care management approaches.

GENERIC ALGORITHMS

Generic algorithms were developed in 1979 and early 1980 at the Rockburn Institute under the direction of Dennis A. Bertram, MD, and Dale N. Schumacher, MD. The algorithm methodology differs from earlier classification approaches in that the purpose for which the classification system is intended dictates the formation of patient groups. Generic algorithms represent an attempt to design a classification system characterized by the following attributes:

- Effectiveness in distinguishing groups in accordance with the purpose of the classification,
- medically meaningful patient groups,
- maximum use of available discharge abstract information, and
- a practical and easily implemented system.

The initial research on generic algorithms focused on the development of medically logical algorithms that would partition a group of patients into categories that are suitable for analyzing resource consumption. The patient groups can be specified by the user; for example, grouping together all patients with a paticular diagnosis or procedure or patients of a certain sex or age. The result of applying the algorithms to a group of patients is the segregation of patients into categories that are both medically meaningful and homogeneous with respect to charges.

The strengths of the generic algorithm approach are:

- it uses all available information on the diagnoses and procedures listed in a discharge abstract;
- it is exhaustive for all diagnostic and procedural codes that could occur on discharge abstracts; and
- it uses an existing hospital data source, the discharge abstract.

The fact that generic algorithms are flexible and base patient groups on variables that reflect characteristics of a specific patient population can be considered either a strength or a weakness, depending on the user's reason for classifying patients. As an internal management tool, flexibility is a strength because the patient groups will reflect the unique patient population served by the institution. However, this characteristic is a weakness if the hospital wants a system with fixed patient categories for purposes of comparison. Another weakness of the methodology is that the algorithms are not sensitive to interactions between diagnoses and procedures (that is, all secondary diagnoses, regardless of their nature, are given equal weighting when combined with a given procedure).

CONCLUSION

With the recent legislation introducing a prospective payment system based on diagnosis related groups, this classification system is receiving much attention. However, diagnosis related groups are just ne of nine very different patient classification systems developed to measure the case mix of health care institutions. The way in which each classification system measures case mix will determine its usefulness in hospital planning, financial, and/or clinical management.

The ability of health care managers to respond to the new per case Medicare limits depends heavily upon data that relate costs to services and services to patients. Specifically, managers must be able to explain changes in costs in terms of both the volume and type of services provided and the cost of producing those services. Changes in the volume of services provided can be attributed to variations in the mix of patients admitted, in the use of routine and ancillary services, and in length of stay. Changes in the cost of producing hospital services can be traced to changes in the productivity of the hospital's human and other resources or to changes in the "prices" of those resources, including wages.

Although cost per case could be used exclusively for coping with the new regulations, its application to all aspects of hospital operations is not only possible, but also preferable. Once developed, the case-mix data base can be used to define the hospital product in terms of a patient-classification scheme. Thus, the case-mix system is not only a means of coping with changes in reimbursement, but also is a way of ensuring health care management's future viability through efficient and effective management techniques.

Putting the DRG prospective method of case-mix reimbursement in its proper perspective as only one of many case-mix approaches affords health care managers several advantages. These include not only developing an understanding of how DRG can be improved, but also of the planning, directing, controlling, and budgeting issues that led to the rise of case mix itself. In order to be able to control and influence, rather than be controlled by the patterns of reform already irrevolcably set into motion, nothing less than such an understanding is acceptable. The choice rests in each health care manager's hands.

WILL YOUR COMPUTER MEET YOUR CASE-MIX INFORMATIONAL NEEDS?

Jane Fedorowicz

Computers have historically played a secondary role in the running of a hospital. In the early days, the computer was viewed as a tool—an aid to the laboratory technician in the testing process, or a mechanized bookkeeping instrument for the billing and payroll department. Little by little, we saw the advent of computerization in other areas of the hospital. Admissions and nurses' schedules were added to the accounting systems, and EKGs were computerized.

Soon, hospitals found that they were purchasing many small computers. Accounting and patient information shared the mainframe computer, but laboratories and other clinical support functions required specialized equipment. Often, these systems were selected by the user departments, with the results being that no coordination or integration would be possible at a later date.

The mandate to base Medicare payments on prospective pricing (using DRGs) will now force hospitals to recognize the importance of integrating their information systems. Case-mix requirements stipulate the use of both medical and patient-care data. Given the scenario described, this task would be close to impossible. Hospitals are now asking: "Short of starting over, can we adapt our information systems to meet the needs of prospective payment?"

The outlook is not as bleak as it appears thus far. Let us begin to answer this question by ascertaining the requirements of a case-mix system.

CASE-MIX REQUIREMENTS

The Medicare prospective-payment system will place new demands on the hospital information system (HIS). Data from the general ledger, medical records, and billing must be combined to unite the diagnosis for a patient with services received and the cost of those services. For the first time, management will have to monitor physician actions and medical record procedures to ensure that the hospital is providing the correct mix of services to its patients and that it is doing so in a cost-efficient manner. What specific changes will this entail?

The major alteration resulting from the new government requirements mandates a change in management philosophy. A hospital has always been run as two separate organizations—the administrators control the finances and resources of the hospital, and the medical organization directs the volume of services provided to the patient. HISs have supported this dichotomy by providing financial and utilization data for management purposes and clinical information to support the medical functions. The change in philosophy results from the need for administrators to manage and control the utilization of resources and the cost of services for the overriding purpose of keeping the hospital solvent. Administrators will need integrated HISs to provide this utilization information.

In addition to the Medicare application, administrators are discovering that case-mix measurements have other uses in the hospital. These classification schemes are being applied to budgeting, planning, utilization review, and quality assurance. The basic requirements for each of these applications are the same: integration of financial and patient data. However, researchers have noted that each use of case-mix classification may require a different set of data, for example, different factors than those used for quality assurance are needed to classify patients for prospective payment schemes. In a study by the Hospital Research and Educational Trust, nine distinct classification schemes were identified.[1] Table 1 lists them, along with the major development objective of each.

The principal factor in most of these schemes is diagnosis (admitting and/or discharge); other important factors include the presence or absence of surgery, type of surgery, complications, comorbidity, severity of illness, age, and type of care. The designer of a case-mix system must be aware that the same set of patient categories may not be appropriate for every application in the hospital. The system can and should be designed to accommodate different uses, especially now that administrators are finding that detailed utilization data are necessary for improving the financial performance of the hospital.

In a special report by the American Hospital Association on the management implications of the changes in Medicare policy, strategies for employing case-mix schemes for better financial management were developed.[2] These include methods for increasing productivity levels and better management of

---

[1] M. F. Plomann, *Nine Patient Classification Schemes: Development, Description, and Testing* (Chicago: The Hospital Research and Education Trust, 1982).

[2] American Hospital Association, "Medicare Payment: Special Report 3, Legislative Summary and Management Implication," *Healthcare Financial Management,* 13(8):47-52, August 1983.

Table 1.
Purpose of Classification of Nine Case-Mix Schemes

Utilization Review	Reimbursement	Quality Assurance	Management
Diagnosis Related Groups ICD-9-CM List A	MD-DADO Patient Management Categories	AS-SCORE Disease Staging Severity-of-Illness Index	Generic Algorithms VA Multi-Level Care Groups

length of stay. Table 2 summarizes the strategies proposed by the AHA.

Parallels to many of these strategies have been employed in the business world for years. Hospital administrators are now encountering the same problems that businesses have always faced: they must learn how to hold costs down in order to stay in business. The key to maintaining control over costs lies in the quality of information available to managers. In this respect, the Medicare proposal forces the manager to improve his access to information. How this is to be accomplished depends on the status of the HIS in place at this time. We turn now to a discussion of currently available HISs.

TRENDS IN HOSPITAL INFORMATION SYSTEMS

Initial attempts at computerization in hospitals led to the proliferation of the independently developed, stand-alone systems described earlier. Ball and Boyle classify these as Class A systems.[3]

Table 2.
Case-Mix Financial Management Strategies

Productivity Improvements	Length-of-Stay Management
Personnel Budgets	Discharge Planning
Inventory Management	Referrals to Other Providers
Utilization Evaluation of Capital, Equipment, and Services	Monitoring/Reductions in Inpatient Service Usage
Capital Investments Analysis	Internal Utilization Review and Quality Assurance Programs

---

[3]M. J. Ball and T. M. Boyle, "Hospital Information Systems: Past, Present, and Future," *Hospital Financial Management*, February 1980, pp. 12-14.

As HISs became more advanced, some integration was introduced, usually based on financial applications. Integration categorizes a system as Class B in Ball and Boyle's terminology. A Class B Level 1 system primarily provides billing support. In these systems, admissions/discharge/transfer (ADT) and order entry interface with the billing system, providing a mechanism for charge capturing. Level 1 systems contain records of patient stay, but do not provide any continuity over time, since they are constructed to accommodate the billing function. Thus, medical records and test results must be maintained separately.

When a Class B system is capable of retaining historical medical record data, it is considered a Level 2 system. When an order is placed, the billing component is updated, and a historical record is the state of the art in HISs today.

Ball and Boyle also describe a Class C system, which is based on the medical record. The crux of this system is medical data rather than financial or administrative data, as in a Class B system. Few of these systems have been implemented, and they are still in the experimental stage.

An HIS can be obtained through three channels. These include time-sharing and shared-service vendors, purchased systems, and inhouse development. All three have been available for more than 20 years.

The price of hardware compels many hospitals to go outside for computer access. Time-sharing and shared-service vendors provide both hardware and software to hospitals. The hospital that cannot afford to purchase a machine or employ the extensive manpower needed to support the data processing function can pay these firms to use their programs and facilities. However, as the price of hardware plummets and HISs are developed for smaller computers, this alternative has become less attractive to even the smaller hospitals.[4,5]

Most medium- to large-sized hospitals have found that the best source of applications software has been the commercial vendor. Hospitals can purchase software for most of their applications from firms specializing in the development of generalized application programs or can commission a vendor to develop a special application.

If a particular application is not available commercially, or if many changes to an off-the-shelf system must be made to render it useful to the hospital, the application may be developed inhouse. This is more time-consuming and more expensive than purchasing a commercially available system and is only recommended for applications that cannot be obtained from a vendor.

In a recent study of Chicago-area hospitals, 30 percent of the hospitals had inhouse hardware only, 35 percent used an outside service vendor, and 35 percent used both inhouse and outside service vendors. For current inhouse users, 35 percent of software programs were modified from a purchased package, 29 percent were developed by the inhouse staff, and 35 percent were developed entirely by outside contractors.[6]

---

[4] "IBM Unveils HIS for Small Hospitals," *Modern Healthcare*, May 1981a, p. 126.

[5] "NCR, H-P Kick Off New HIS Plans," *Modern Healthcare*, May 1981b, pp. 118-120.

[6] Hospital Financial Management Association, *Data Processing Information Survey: Chicago Area Hospitals* (Oak Brook, IL: HFMA, First Illinois Chapter, 1981).

The Chicago hospitals were also asked to estimate the percentage of total data processing services used by their financial, clinical, and administrative functions. The response demonstrates hospitals' orientation toward computerizing financial and administrative tasks: financial applications made up 73.8 percent of all data processing performed; clinical functions, 12.6 percent; administrative/statistics, 11.4 percent; and other, the remaining 2.2 percent.

Many of these financial applications are needed for a case-mix payment scheme; however, a true management tool requires the integration of clinical and patient information, found only in Level 2 or Class C systems. Unfortunately, most hospitals do not have these types of systems. Jacobs surveyed U.S. hospitals and found that, of those with more than 50 beds, 98 percent have computerized business and financial systems, in-hospital or shared. Approximately 700 of the 4,800 U.S. short-term hospitals have installed Level 1 HISs. Approximately 200 have installed Level 2 HISs.[7]

Recent announcements of Level 2 systems' availability on small computers should alleviate this somewhat. These new systems should make HISs affordable to smaller hospitals, which had been left behind because of the high cost of large-scale integrated systems.

HIS APPLICATIONS

The number and sophistication of HIS applications vary greatly across hospitals and vendors, whether or not they are considered Class A or Class B systems. Inevitably, however, hospitals tend to computerize laboratory and financial applications early on, following these with administrative and other support functions.[8] This observation is supported by the HFMA study, which included a survey of computerized applications in the 77 responding hospitals.[9] The responses indicate that most of these hospitals do not have a fully integrated HIS that could provide the comprehensive set of information needed for a case-mix system capable of monitoring costs and services to the hospital. According to Kukla and Bachofer, the HIS will need " . . . to provide information on the types of patients admitted to the hospital and the types of services offered to patients during their hospital stay. They also will be equipped to handle more sophisticated analysis of those factors that determine the total cost of hospital services, including the volume of services produced, productivity of resources used, and price of resources. In addition, hospitals will develop greater sophistication in forecasting cost and utilization."[10]

---

[7]S.E. Jacobs, "Hospital-wide Computer Systems: The Market and the Vendors," *MUG Quarterly*, 12(3):1-12, Fall 1982

[8]T.R. Prince and J. Fedorowicz, "Hospital Information Systems Development Patterns," presented at TIMS/ORSA Joint National Meeting, Chicago, April 1983.

[9]Hospital Financial Management Association, *op. cit.*

[10]S.F. Kukla and H.J. Bachofer, "Building Up Reporting Systems, *Hospitals*, 57(14):79, July 16, 1983.

Table 3.
1981 HFMA Survey Results

Application Area	Totally Manual	Automated	System Status within 1 Year	1-3 Years	Total Responses
Administrative					
Key Factor Performance Statistics	24	24	6	12	66
Forecasting/Simulation	27	15	7	14	63
Admissions					
Patient Information Collection	4	54	8	9	75
Patient Transfers and Discharge	5	58	8	6	77
Business Office					
Inpatient Billing	1	66	5	4	76
Medicare/Medicaid Reporting	18	44	6	4	72
Financial Analysis of Department Performances	7	54	7	6	74
Annual Budget Preparation	16	43	8	8	75
Exception Reporting of Performance Analysis	25	33	6	7	71
Rate Setting	37	16	6	10	69
Clinical Laboratory/Pathology					
Daily Log of Tests Requested	28	22	11	11	72
Online Data Acquisition	22	23	11	10	66
Charge Capturing	20	35	9	10	74

Application Area	Totally Manual	Automated	System Status within 1 Year	1–3 Years	Total Responses
Radiological Services					
Results Reporting	44	7	7	14	72
Medical Areas—Common Functions					
Order Entry	34	18	6	16	74
Results Reporting	40	9	5	19	73
Progress Reports (observations, diagnoses)	48	5	1	17	71
Interdepartmental Communications	47	10	4	11	72
Medical Records					
Patient-Number Retrieval	25	23	13	10	70
Disease Index	28	24	5	14	71
Patient-Record Storage and Retrieval	49	9	5	11	74
Utilization Review	40	12	5	14	71
Nursing Services					
Results Reporting and Chart Preparation	47	9	3	16	75
Staffing and Patient-Load Records	50	5	6	13	74
Pharmacy					
Filling Medication Orders	35	18	11	12	76
Patient Drug Profiles	26	23	13	11	73

These capabilities imply that the HIS will be an integrated system providing on-line entry and retrieval of all patient-related service data in the hospital. The requirements of case-mix also imply that the HIS maintain a high level of reliability in the content and completeness of its data base. Where do hospitals stand relative to the requirements of such a system?

To answer this, let us examine some of the results of the Chicago HFMA survey. Respondents were asked to indicate whether each application area (in a list of 95) was performed manually or on the computer, or if plans for automation were approved for implementation in the near future. A subset of 26 applications that are considered representative of the applications needed for case-mix construction are contained in Table 3.

The survey shows that most (but not all) of the hospitals have computerized their admissions and billing functions, which are two of the sources of data required in a case-mix application.

Smaller numbers of hospitals have financial and administrative support for management tasks of budgeting and planning. The laboratory and pharmacy are somewhat automated, although they probably use a stand-alone minicomputer in many hospitals. The remaining necessary applications are computerized in only a small percentage of the responding hospitals.

Medical records and ancillary services remain manual systems in the majority of these hospitals. Two-thirds of the hospitals do not plan on implementing interdepartmental communications in their medical areas in the foreseeable future. Applications such as nurse staffing, which should be part of the planning function, are also not computerized. The bottom line is that very few hospitals will *easily* be able to adapt their present HIS to a full-fledged case-mix payment and planning system.

CASE-MIX IMPLEMENTATION

An estimated two years of development time may be required to set up a cost-accounting system for case-mix analysis.[11] Many data processing departments anticipated the new Medicare requirements and began development ahead of time.

One of the first uses of the cost-accounting data produced by a case-mix system should be to verify the case-mix index (CMI) assigned to the hospital by HCFA. A retrospective study of 1980 Medicare billings, on which CMIs are based, could lead to a higher index (and, therefore, higher revenue). Additional benefits may also be incurred by this activity. Rodney Klein of the Jewish Hospital of St. Louis discusses these benefits: "You develop a profile by physician and product line, at least on the revenue side. You can pinpoint trends and get valuable management and marketing information by going back to 1980."[12]

[11] "Strategies for Change," *Hospitals,* 57(13):58-63, July 1, 1983.

[12] *Ibid.,* p. 60.

The retrospective studies can be coupled with demographic information to provide the manager with forecasts of the changing service requirements of a shifting population. As can be imagined, this type of system will require data from many computer files. Let us examine some alternative sources of data and processing.

Shared-service vendors comprise one source of case-mix applications. Typically, service is limited to Medicare billing and DRG computation. Advanced applications for cost accounting and planning purposes are not yet available through this outlet. However, these shared-services can be used to fill the gap until a tailored system is introduced into the hospital.

Some commercial vendors have incorporated DRG analysis into their HISs. Hospitals currently using their systems can add on a module for the new billing system. Again, these systems provide the minimum analysis, and sophisticated decision support is not yet available.

Inhouse development or contracting with consultants are the only currently feasible alternatives to providing the decision-support capabilities that administrators want and need. There are ways of providing this support. One is to use the hospital-wide data base and computer system, and the other is to "down-load" needed data to a microcomputer for the administrator's use. Both have their advantages.

The degree of difficulty in accessing an HIS for the new application depends upon the way in which the data are stored. Many HISs are "file-based"; each application has its own file containing all of the data needed to run its programs. If more than one application uses overlapping pieces of data (for example, patient name and number), these are replicated in each file. When a new application is to be developed with new data requirements, new files are created. In order for an administrator to access the data stored in this way, the application will be limited to accessing data currently stored, or new files will have to be constructed. Both require a great deal of development time. Some hospitals circumvent the problems of a file-based system by manually computing and/or entering DRGs to the Medicare billing system. This shortcut method should be only an interim step until a better system can be implemented.

Many hospitals have replaced their file-based systems with data-base technology. A data-base management system (DBMS) is a collection of interrelated data that can be used by many applications through a common base of software. DBMS software adds great flexibility to an HIS, enabling changes to be made to the data base or to the programs' accessing it with less effort and less expense than in file-oriented systems. DBMS technology is used in some, but not all, Level 2 and Class C systems. A DBMS provides the level of integration needed for obtaining accurate cost information.[13] In addition, most have a user-oriented query facility that allows the nonprogramming user

---

[13] J. Fedorowicz and S. Veazie, "Automated DRG Systems: Unanswered Questions," *Hospital Progress,* 6(1):54-55,71, January 1981.

to access and manipulate the data base. It is this query language that would enable the administrator to directly ask planning-related questions of the system without having to wait for a program to be written. One caution should be noted here: query languages require a great deal of system time and overhead, taking away computational power from other applications using the data base. Care should be taken that normal hospital processing does not suffer due to its overuse.

This caution is one of the main reasons for providing the administrator with a microcomputer (and it applies to a file-based system, as well). Historical usage data can be copied to a microcomputer, freeing up valuable mainframe time. The micro user has the full use of the system and its data, and can manipulate it in any way without affecting other hospital users. New, easy-to-use software, including decision-support systems, spread-sheet analysis, and word-processing programs, render the micro accessible for most uses. These systems are cheaper than their mainframe counterparts; their major limitations are the smaller amount of data that can be accessed and their slower manipulation speed.

All of these technologies can be used to derive different case-mix constructs for the diverse objectives of a particular hospital. Obviously, a DBMS or microcomputer will simplify the process, but file-based systems are also feasible. The key problem is whether or not all of the requisite data are being collected, and, if so, whether they are accessible in the form needed by the case-mix programs. An equally important issue concerns the reliability of the data. The old adage, "garbage in, garbage out," is especially important when all the data upon which decisions are based are stored in the computer.

CONCLUSION

Hospitals lag behind their corporate counterparts in the sophistication of their computer systems. Much information in hospitals is still processed manually, and that which is computerized is not always accessible in the format or combination needed. When faced with case-mix requirements, hospitals are finding that automation and integration of information are imperative. Improved cost-accounting systems must be developed in order for a hospital to survive in an increasingly competitive industry.

RELATIVE INTENSITY MEASURES AND THE STATE OF THE ART OF REIMBURSEMENT FOR NURSING SERVICES

Lucille A. Joel

CASE MIX, RATE SETTING, AND REIMBURSEMENT

A case mix is no more than a taxonomy or classification system, a way of organizing observations of reality according to select principles that increase the predictive efficiency of the information. Diagnosis related groups (DRGs) are a classification system of patients grouped according to their hospital resource use. This system was originally developed at Yale University through the pioneering work of John Thompson, a nurse and researcher.

Thompson's intent was to create a model for peer review of physicians that would characterize usual or reasonable clinical management practices. Through the process of factor analysis, homogeneous categories were constructed that cluster cases according to hospital resource use. The resources in question are 1) length of stay and 2) diagnostic and therapeutic ancillary services. Both of these factors are accessed to patients through physician prescription; hence, the link to peer review. The independent variables, or clinical characteristics, that were the significant determinants of resource consumption became the organizational elements of the classification system. These variables are: 1) primary diagnosis, 2) the presence or absence of surgery and complications, 3) secondary diagnosis, and 4) age. After a period of trial and incorporation into rate setting in the state of New Jersey, the original classification system was refined to include 23 major diagnosis related groups (DRGs).

Using the statistical technique of regression, a variance for each DRG was established. Ideally, 95 percent of the cases categorized within the DRG will consume an amount of resources within the parameters of the variance. It can be statistically assumed that, by pure chance, 5 percent of the cases included in a DRG will use either more or fewer resources than the predicted limits. The variance, or parameters, of predicted resource use are described in terms of a range for the length of stay. There is a basic premise that consumption of diagnostic and therapeutic ancillary services is in some way proportionate

57

to the length of stay. The range of the usual length of stay is called the *trim point.* Patients falling outside this range are *outliers.* The billing for outliers is based on controlled charges, while hospitals are reimbursed an all-inclusive dollar amount for the aggregate services delivered to a patient who falls within the variance. This amount differs with each DRG.

The social mandate to curtail escalating health care costs preceded DRGs, as did the realization that the major offenders within this costly conspiracy were hospitals. Given the capacity of the DRG system to predict and quantify hospital resource use and the relationship of resource use to cost, it was natural to effect a marriage between DRGs and reimbursement.

Through analysis of a hospital's historical patient population, predictions can be made concerning the nature and extent of resources that will be necessary for a forthcoming budget period. In rate-setting jargon, the case mix profile in the base year can be used to budget prospectively. Assuming no major shifts in case mix, the resources necessary for each department can be fairly well detailed. Budgetary increases resolve around trending the base year forward, based on inflation and other economic factors. The ultimate end of controlling overall cost is achieved through fixing each departmental cost center, based on historical patterns of use. This technique also has an impact on the practice of cross-subsidization between departments. Traditionally, the charge to the patient for services in high-volume departments has been substantially greater than actual cost in order to generate revenue and to offset the deficits sustained through less frequently used or extremely costly areas.

Hospitals will become increasingly comfortable with the predictive efficiency of the system as they institute more cost-efficient management and shape the ordering practices of physicians. To promote conforming behaviors, an incentive system has been designed to "sweeten the pot." Where the actual cost of the patient's hospital episode is less than the inclusive amount for the DRG, the hospital may keep the difference. This same psychology of shaping and conformity is obvious in the establishment of rates. Both the New Jersey and Medicare methodologies aim to eventually base rates fully on a state or national standard. Simply put, a hospital's rate is currently a combination of the actual cost to the institution and of a standard established through digesting information on a larger scale. Initially, the rate is blended generously in favor of the hospital's own cost. Each successive computation increases the proportion in favor of the standard. By 1987, Medicare rates will be fully standardized, with the only differences being between rural and urban hospitals.

THE ISSUE: RELATIVE INTENSITY
MEASURES OF NURSING (RIMs)

Both the New Jersey and Medicare reimbursement systems share one common characteristic: the manner in which nursing resource use is costed. Nursing is included in the *per diem* calculation and is therefore inextricably bound to the length of stay. There is no appreciation of the variability of nursing resource use from patient to patient. While the cost of nursing is averaged and dispersed equally among all patients, there is little possibility of predicting and controlling that portion of the institutional budget that represents nursing. This becomes a serious issue, since the basic approach to cost curtailment is budget control on a department-to-department basis. In most situations, nursing represents 35 to 50 percent of the hospital budget.

This historical manner of costing out our services has seriously retarded nursing's growth as a profession. The anonymity of the per-diem charge has devalued our service and created major consumer inequities. Even the most unsophisticated eye can see that every hospitalized patient neither needs nor gets the same amount of nursing service. The absence of patient-specific measures of nursing resource use has promoted the phenomena of cross-subsidization and down-substitution. Because their service could not be quantified, nurses have been made to perform nonnursing activities, including activities below their skill level. The rape of the nursing budget has been through manpower drain rather than dollar drain.

In 1977, the New Jersey Department of Health initiated a contract with the federal government's Health Care Financing Administration, promising that by 1982 it would have developed a nursing resource allocation model that is DRG-specific. The department exceeded its expectation and has generated a separate case mix that quantifies nursing resource use on a patient-specific basis and has then conveniently linked these computations to DRGs for ease in billing. In order to establish the credibility of this system, which had its genesis in New Jersey, it is necessary to go back to the research underlying these relative intensity measures of nursing (RIMs) and the methodology through which they are incorporated into rate setting.

The RIMs methodology is the product of a series of studies, the first of which were designed to perfect instrumentation and methodology. It is very worthwhile to look at the results of that early research before going further. Early studies showed a negative correlation between age and nursing resource use. In other words, the older the patient, the fewer nursing resources consumed or provided. This finding proved very controversial and was used to argue against the once-existing 8.5 percent Medicare nursing differential. The issue of whether the aged consume more nursing resources becomes moot within the current DRG system, since one of the major clinical variables is age. In other words, there are routine corrections for age, eliminating the issue of a differential. Another early study identified a proxy relationship between nursing and nonnursing: as the amount of nursing support services increased, so did the amount of nursing consumed by patients. Conversely, with a decrease in services supportive to nursing, the amount of nursing resource use per patient also decreased. To put it bluntly, where there was no one available to do something, nurses did it.

In eight New Jersey hospitals surveyed during 1979, 38 percent of the resources of the nursing department were invested in nonnursing activities and only 62 percent in nursing activities. This phenomenon can be easily quantified: of a total nursing budget of more than $51,000,000 among these study hospitals, $19,500,000 were invested in nonnursing activities and only $31,500,000 in nursing activities. The greatest cross-subsidization was observed in obstetrics, where 47 percent of the nurses' time was invested in nonnursing activities, and the least in psychiatry, where 26 percent of activities were nonnursing.[1] It should be noted that the classification of an activity as nursing or nonnursing was totally dependent on the judgment of the nurse. An activity could be classified as nonnursing under some circumstances and as nursing under others. A good example is transport. Where the physical or psychosocial condition of the patient warranted a nurse to accompany the patient, the activity was categorized as nursing. When transport could have been safely and therapeutically effected without a nurse, but nurses had to accomplish the task by default, it was classified as nonnursing. The final study to develop statistical equations for hospital nursing resource allocation on a patient-specific basis involved sample of 3,335 patients and 63,400 shifts in eight study hospitals. For each encounter with a patient, the nurse identified a nursing diagnosis, the specific nursing activity performed, the acuity of the nursing diagnosis, and the amount of time consumed.[2] Although a great deal of very rich and relevant nursing information was collected, only the amount of time invested in care was used in the construction of the allocation statistics. This is admittedly a weakness of the methodology. It is debatable whether nursing resource investment can be measured along the single dimension of time. Time represents only one overt measure of the service, but other elements may better characterize the quantitative investment. Financial constraints on the study did not allow using this broader data base in final calculations. Plans for additional grantsmanship are in process, which would allow refinement of RIMs through analysis of the remaining data. It has been the conviction of organized nursing in New Jersey that RIMs deserve the same opportunity for expansion and refinement accorded to DRGs in their early period of development; we have no reason to believe that this courtesy will not be accorded. RIMs were incorporated into New Jersey rate setting on an experimental basis in January of 1984. The precedent has been set; nursing will emerge as a distinct cost center with patient-to-patient variations.

THE METHODOLOGY: RELATIVE INTENSITY MEASURES OF NURSING (RIMs)

A relative intensity measure of nursing is an arithmetic abstraction that serves

---

[1] New Jersey Department of Health, *A Prospective Reimbursement System Based on Patient Case Mix for New Jersey Hospitals, 1976-1983.* Second Annual Report, Volume I (Trenton: State of New Jersey Department of Health, December 1978).

[2] New Jersey Department of Health. *A Prospective Reimbursement System Based on Patient Case Mix for New Jersey Hospitals, 1976-1983, Case Mix Performance Study, Instruction Manual* (Trenton: State of New Jersey Department of Health, September 1979).

Figure 1. Allocating Relative Intensity Measures
(RIMs) to Case Mix Categories

Step 1 **Computing the cost of a RIM**

$$\frac{\text{Total actual nursing cost: } \$14,000,000}{\text{Total minutes of nursing resource use: } 112,000,000 \text{ minutes}} = 12\frac{1}{2}\text{¢ per RIM}$$

(A RIM is actually 1 minute of nursing resource use)

Step 2 **Computing the number of RIMs per case**

A. Employing algorithm or decision tree, assign each case to a Nursing Research Cluster (NRC).

B. Select appropriate equation from among NRC equations to calculate number of RIMs per case.

Step 3 **Computing average nursing intensity per DRG**

A. Assign each case to its DRG.

B. Average RIMs for all patients within DRG and assign cost.

Example: DRG 369   Patient 1—1800 RIMs @ 12½¢ each = 225
Patient 2—1200 RIMs @ 12½¢ each = 150
Patient 3— 900 RIMs @ 12½¢ each = 112.50
Patient 4— 800 RIMs @ 12½¢ each = 100
Patient 5—1700 RIMs @ 12½¢ each = 212.50
Patient 6—1000 RIMs @ 12½¢ each = 125

Total 7400 RIMs @ 12½¢ each = $925.00

925 ÷ 6 patients = Average nursing cost per case, or $154.17

as a proxy for charges in describing nursing resource use. (The calculation process is detailed in Figure 1.) The process involves three phases: identifying the cost of a RIM, determining the number of RIMs per case, and calculating the average nursing resource use within each DRG. Simply put, the cost per RIM is the relationship between the total actual cost of nursing in the institution and the number of minutes of nursing time used by the recipients of care. One RIM equals one minute. A RIM may be more or less costly, depending upon the skill mix of nursing staff, with more skilled personnel receiving higher salaries. Primary nursing should reflect a more costly RIM, but this remains an internal decision. RIMs preserve the management prerogatives within each hospital.

The second phase of the cost-allocation process involves assigning the appropriate number of RIMs to each case in the base year. Ideally, this base year is the one preceding the year for which rates will be prospectively computed. Contiguous years provide the greatest comparability in case mix. RIMs per case are computed through a two-step decision-making process. First, each case is assigned to a nursing resource cluster (NRC). Then, one of several equations existing within the NRC is applied to the patient-specific data. The NRCs and equations are the analogs of MDCs and DRGs. Their organization reflects the variables that were most predictive of the intensity of nursing resource use. Those variables were limited by virtue of the data that were analyzed. Primary diagnosis was the major independent variable, with admission and discharge status, length of stay, and the presence or absence of surgery offering additional significant projections.

Each case is finally assigned to a DRG category in order to establish an average cost of nursing for the DRG. It should be noted that, hypothetically, each patient within a DRG may have had RIMs calculated through a different NRC or equation.

The RIMs allocation statistics will change as nursing changes. New Jersey nursing has proposed an oversight committee of representatives from both the profession and the hospital industry to monitor changes in practice. The individual institutional budget for nursing should vary according to yearly changes in the case mix and the numbers of nursing-intensive patients. Without a nursing allocation model, there is no way to document what patients are nursing-intensive *versus* ancillary-intensive.

RIMs should be judged on what they are, not on what they are not. **RIMs are relative, not absolute.** They merely provide a methodology to more equitably divide the cost of nursing among the patient population. They do not increase the dollar amount of the nursing budget, although management information accessed through RIMs can be used to build a case for increased demands on the nursing department. **RIMs are not a staffing tool.** They provide an aggregate, interval measure of resource consumption. Day-to-day, ordinal measures are still necessary to staffing decisions. **RIMs are not a measure of pure nursing.** They measure the relative consumption of the resources of nursing among the patients. If the nursing department chooses to have nurses engage in nonnursing activities, that is an internal decision. New Jersey nurses have chosen the regulatory route to have their service emerge as a cost center in hospitals. They propose neither this approach nor the RIMs methodology as necessarily the route for the profession beyond their state.

RIMS are not perfect. We offer them for your review while being fully aware of their imperfections. However, any criticism is dwarfed by the benefits that they promise to hospitals and to the profession. We realize that the data necessary to establish a credible standard are not currently available and that our state computer system is straining under the massive data that must be processed. A grievance-and-appeal system exists, but it is inefficient, cumbersome, and slow; management reports generated through this system leave much to be desired. Despite all this, we can verify that RIMs are more refined than DRGs were upon their introduction into rate setting. It is more dangerous to remain anonymous that to cast our lot with the beginning system.

GEARING UP FOR DRGs

Though RIMs may only be of academic interest to most of the profession, the need to "gear up" for DRGs has become personally meaningful since October 1983. Some observations from the history of a state where DRG-based reimbursement was phased in over three years may be useful.

Hospitals successful in competing in this new world of reimbursement become characterized by a short length of stay, high volume, and a complex case mix. This complex case mix is predictably nursing-intensive. Diagnosis and treatment of the medical problem and stablization of the treatment regime can be accomplished quite expeditiously in these times. Much medical management can even be conducted comfortably through ambulatory or community services. Patients who have an extended length of stay and are therefore costly more often reflect nursing needs rather than medical needs. Primary concerns become the development of community and family support systems, teaching, counseling, and functional ability and self-care. The fact that so many of these costly patients are nursing-intensive and that, on the whole, all patients will display a greater level of acuity predicts that more nursing manpower will be needed to do the job for the same daily census of patients. A serious manpower shortfall seems unavoidable; yet there is no proof of change in total nursing resource consumption. The frightening alternative may be to break up costly professional lines to fund a large number of less-skilled hands to do the job. The outcome could be a work environment where there is less time than ever to nurse, less job satisfaction, lower-level clinical nursing services and, consequently, even greater problems with recruitment and retention than we have experienced to date.

The secret to survival in these times is the creation and management of information, innovative use of human resources, and assertive action to establish the practice autonomy of nursing in hospitals. These elements are not presented in any operational sequence; rather, activity in one area is both basic to, and builds on, the others. A good place to begin is to admit that we live in an informational age. Further, a distinction must be made between internal and external data. RIMs provide New Jersey nurses with both internal and interagency data.

Interagency comparisons are currently inadequate due to vast differences in nursing among practice sites in the state and to the quality of the data that come to the state from some hospitals. The internal data hold great possibility and can lend direction for seeking more detailed information about specific hospital units or providers. The informational capacity of RIMs can be provided through other strategies. Somehow, nursing's resource use has to be reduced to a patient-specific level in order to successfully compete with the precedent set by DRGs. Changes in case mix and related resource consumption have to be monitored, and evidence must accrue to prove nursing's contribution to institutional fiscal solvency.

One should begin by identifying which cases are most costly in terms of nursing, why they are costly, the volume of those cases, and the percent of total volume that they represent. This can be accomplished by judiciously making use of the data that have been generated in New Jersey or through agency-specific information, or can be based upon expert opinion. Once these data have been summarized, clinical nursing consultation should be sought so as to maximize the therapeutic effectiveness and cost efficiency of care to these populations. This could be the opportunity to turn turmoil into triumph and establish a renewed mutual respect between nurse administrators and clinicians. Sophisticated clinicians hold the secret to decreasing lengths of stay, avoiding complications, and reducing the use of diagnostic and therapeutic ancillary services. More precision and sophistication in the documentation of clinical nursing can, in and of itself, have an impact on physician ordering patterns. Nurse managers must be open to ideas for geographic reorganization and regionalization based on the nursing needs of patients and the availability of clinical skill. They must encourage control of practice through such institutional mechanisms as nursing staff organizations, practice councils, and peer-review models. Demonstration and pilot projects should be designed that incorporate creative skill mix and staffing patterns.

In summary, hospitals are the prime employment arena for most nurses. There is no hope for autonomy unless we begin to quantify our contribution. Reimbursement methodology and cost-containment pressures can offer an opportunity, rather than an obstacle, to our progress. All professional providers are under obligation to develop to new awareness of the relationship between cost, cure, and care, and to modify their approach to practice accordingly. Nurses have always been central to the coordination of care in hospitals and have been the "fine-tuners" at the unit level. These new circumstances promise an opportunity for us to demonstrate our contribution and move on to controlling our own practice.

A NURSING PERSPECTIVE OF THE DRG WORLD

Franklin A. Shaffer

While federal officials' longstanding concern and action with regard to soaring Medicare spending is no longer news, the rapid development and scope of their actions require our continued close attention and reeducation. The change continues to advance upon us relentlessly, oblivious to whether or not we understand the ramifications of its power to affect us. Whether we choose to make the effort to understand how this ongoing transition will change our careers will determine the future of nursing as a profession.

It is the purpose of this paper to present an overview of the recent developments that have created the changes that we face, not merely to survive the present changes, but also to take advantage of them to move forward to higher levels of responsibility. Indeed, the newest changes in Medicare reimbursement offer possibilities both for growth and for decline in the vitality of nursing as a profession. It is up to us to use the opportunities that have been opened to us both to increase our understanding and to make ourselves heard as a convincing voice for increasing quality without increasing cost in care.

LEGISLATIVE REVIEW

To review: In April, 1983, President Reagan signed Public Law (P.L.) 98-21, the Social Security Amendments of 1983. It should be emphasized again that Title VI of this law changes the way that Medicare determines how much hospitals are reimbursed for inpatient care. Federal officials believe that these changes will pare escalating Medicare spending, and thereby alleviate forecasted deficits in the Hospital Insurance Trust Fund of the Social Security program. Indeed, the *Federal Register* of September 1, 1983, published interim final rules, implementing Medicare's new plan, for use in setting payment rates. Further developments enforcing cost-cutting measures are forthcoming.

In the past, Medicare reimbursed hospitals according to the reasonable cost of services rendered to its beneficiaries. This billing was done *retrospectively*, after services were rendered. Hospitals were thus paid a per diem rate for both routine and special care and cost for each ancillary service. The inflationary nature of this method lies in its tendency to discourage efficient provision of health care. The system, in short, encourages hospitals to continue to provide services as long as revenue—in the form of Medicare reimbursement—is maximized.

PROSPECTIVE PAYMENT SYSTEM UPDATE:
HOW IT IS HAPPENING

The new payment system will be phased in gradually over a three-year period, with all elements in place within four years. The way that it will work involves the following factors:

1. HCFA sets limits on how much each hospital can be paid for each DRG.

2. For the first year these limits are based prinicipally on the hospital's *own base year costs;* gradually this will be *completely switched to national averages.* In other words, within four years hospitals will bill exclusively on the basis of what the federal government determines to be the national averages for each diagnosis. We are living, then, in a transitional era, heading rapidly for the reimbursement according to nationally determined ceilings on medical diagnosis prospective billing irrespective of what an individual hospital spends to treat patients.

3. How, then, does the federal government determine what each hospital's reimbursement rate shall be? As mentioned immediately above, it must be understood that the computation breaks down into two sections: the federal government's portion (determined as an across-the-board figure for all hospitals receiving Medicare reimbursement, regardless of individual variation) and the individual hospital's portion (determined according to factors based on the individual hospital resource consumption relating to unique hospital needs). As time progresses, that is, within four years, the system will increasingly impose limits on the basis of the federal government's portion and less on the basis of the individual hospital's portion. And as this process accelerates, cost limits will correspondingly grow more unyielding to individual variation because these differences in hospital resource consumption will be presumed by the federal monitoring system to have been incorporated in the current interim period.

CORDT: THE FEDERAL GOVERNMENT'S SYSTEM
FOR MONITORING ABUSE

While many nursing professionals have expressed concern to the contrary, efforts to function efficiently are not inevitably inconsistent with the goal of rendering quality care. Indeed, if specific tests and procedures have not been furnished efficiently, or if certain diseases have not been treated in the least costly manner, eliminating these inefficiencies may not impair quality. Rather, the savings can supply more and better services. Reducing unnecessary services to patients will also contribute to cost reduction without quality impairment. Specialization will further encourage high volume treatment of conditions in hospitals best suited to provide it.

A brief understanding of the measures that the federal government is adopting to enforce quality control will be helpful. This will help to reinforce this paper's principal theme that we *must* work together to gear up for these changes. Tucked away in an office in HCFA's Baltimore headquarters is the nucleus of a nationwide network of computers to track hospitals' every move under the prospective payment system. This will enable HCFA, its regional offices, and, soon, fiscal intermediaries, to keep close watch on the hospitals covered by the Medicare payment system. The "Central Office and Regional Dispersal Terminal Network" (CORDT) will enable HCFA to have the necessary data to prove or disprove that proprietary hospitals will make a windfall profit under the prospective payment system (PPS).[1] This will be accomplished by monitoring a hospital's case-mix history. Indeed, the centerpiece of the CORDT system is admission pattern monitoring (APM), which is CORDT's most effective means to detect admission abuses. It is more than a policing system. Like the diagnosis related groups (DRGs) system on which it is based, CORDT is also a tool that can streamline management in the hospitals on the system. But let us understand some of the details of the CORDT system.

Approximately 1,500 hospitals are currently under the HCFA prospective payment system and they are monitored by CORDT. Further, all individual acute care hospitals will be on the prospective payment system network by the fiscal year 1984. The CORDT network monitors every readmission that takes place within seven days of discharge with the rationale that this kind of return of patients for further treatment tends to avoid cost ceilings as they are currently imposed. Other cost-increasing activities monitored are transfers from acute-care units to distinct units that are excluded from the prospective payment system's ceilings. These are watched closely by CORDT in each hospital on the system.

In addition, all transfers from prospective payment system hospitals to those still based on cost-based reimbursement will be closely monitored to prevent avoidance of payment ceilings. As a further measure, five percent of all admissions will be sampled randomly by the CORDT system to determine whether services are necessary and appropriate. All day and cost outliers will be watched for their tendency to avoid cost ceilings. Also, all permanent insertions of pacemakers, as well as all other surgical procedures, will be closely scrutinized for possible misclassification of other less costly operations in these high-level reimbursement slots.

---

[1]M.L. Robinson, "Special Report: HCFA's Computerized PPS," *Prospective Payment Guide*, U.S. Government Printing Office, 1(3):5, November 1983.

More detail here with regard to APM will help to clarify the degree to which this system will be able effectively to enforce the prospective payment system. Admissions pattern monitoring involves entering data generated from reviews of hospital admissions records by the professional standards review organization (PSRO/PRO) or the fiscal intermediary. These data are fed into an IBM 4341 computer located in Baltimore. Together, they present a profile of each hospital, which can be compared with the hospital's previous history. It can also be compared with other hospitals in the various regions, the states, and nationwide. If hospitals are found to have questionable admissions patterns, APM triggers a corrective action program. Professional standards review organizations or fiscal intermediaries discuss educational activities designed to correct the questionable admissions patterns. In addition, the PSRO/PRO or intermediary intensifies its review of all of the hospital's future admissions, focusing on specific diagnoses or physician cases. These intensifications may even involve preadmission reviews as well as payments for inappropriate admissions. The most punitive step is civil monetary penalties, which may be imposed on the hospital with questionable admissions practices.

IMPLICATIONS FOR NURSING

Even a reduction in nursing staff need not mean a reduction in quality. One of the steps being taken across the country is to reduce nursing staff. This includes reductions in continuing education, nursing research, and general staff reduction. Some of this staff reduction is being conducted because of concern for the new system, while some of it is being conducted because of the actual reduction of patient census. There is, however, the reverse side to this restaffing pattern in the IV therapy teams that are being disbanded, where nurses are taking over these and other functions. For this reason, continuing education is being developed at unit levels. This theme of reeducation and watchfulness for new opportunities as the system dynamically unfolds can be applied in many of the work areas currently dominated by other professionals, and nursing will be assigned according to its capability at managerial efficiency.

The beginning of an understanding of the importance of nursing's role in management is its ability to interpret and apply the data that will become increasingly available in management information reports. The prospective payment system, based on DRGs, brings clinical and financial data together. The problem in the past has been that this kind of relational data base has been limited. Hospitals will increasingly develop their own reports, they will contract with vendors to purchase them, or they will buy the development systems from other hospitals. Many computer packages that develop these reports are not nursing-specific—they do not compute nursing's consumption or allocation of resources according to the intensity relating to each case. Thus, even if nursing becomes more productive, this efficiency is still credited to the hospital's overhead reduction rather than to the management effort made with nursing functions.

Attempts to change this have centered around New Jersey's relative intensity measures (RIMs) method, which attempts to quantify the time spent on patient care according to DRG category. It assigns relative values to this time to determine the cost of each category *for nursing*. But in order to move the current system closer to one that accurately reimburses hospitals and, in turn, nursing, for the work actually performed, other systems should also be studied.

Eventually nurses will have to conceptualize their work according to categories formulated by what Piper has called dependency criteria.[2] These measure the degree to which the patient actually depends upon the nurse for care during the stay in the hospital. The improvement of this system upon the RIM system is that it would induce improvements in actual care quality by tagging nursing care to patient need rather than to actual resources consumed — the characteristic of the RIM system.

The three types of functions presented by Piper are unit specific, DRG specific, and function specific. These activity classifications would thus distinguish purely administrative and purely clinical functions, emphasizing both categories as important for computation of the kind of cost that nursing incurs and the contribution that it makes to the hospital product. Further, this would be accomplished without sacrificing patient care; to the contrary, it would more closely follow patient need as the determinant of nursing care allocation.

There are many organizational changes that are gradually falling into place as a result of the new system. The most prominent of these is participative management and decentralization. There is a movement downward in allocation of nursing management authority. The head nurse and first-line managers become much more important because they control allocation of nursing resources. If these individuals have the information based on the case and cost per case, and cost and utilization of resources per case, they can become more cost conscious and therefore productive in allocating nursing resources. The head nurse is, then, in a pivotal position to control cost.

Because of this decentralization of authority, nursing must enhance its collaboration with medical records; the medical record is the newly appointed financial record of today. Nursing must work out a good relationship with the medical records department to assign staff correctly. Either medical records personnel or nursing personnel may be responsible for accurate record keeping, but *who does what* must be firmly established, and the personnel responsible must be checked to determine whether the information recorded is accurate.

Nurse managers are the vital links between quality and cost because they alone are in contact with the patients 7 days a week, 24 hours a day. The nursing department is the competitive edge for the hospital's public relations on a 24-hour basis. Nurse executives must learn that their staffs can no longer afford to be all things to all people at all times. They must develop a marketing plan for the products they offer to the community. As competition increases, patients will be drawn by the quality of care. Nurses have to understand

---

[2]L.P. Piper, "Accounting for Nursing Function in DRGs," *Nursing Management,* 14:(11):44-48, November 1983.

how valuable the client contact is in such a marketing approach.

In addition, there is an opportunity for nursing and other hospital management to establish closer ties. This includes both medical staff and financial staff. Physicians, heretofore excluded from the financial management of the hospitals, are being employed as medical directors — as part of the top management team. Nursing managers will be working more closely with the physicians and financial administrative team, as well as with the medical records department.

In the course of these transformations of the hospital organizational structure, nurse administrators must begin to understand, by continually monitoring the management information reports, what variables influence cost and to keep these under control. By providing precise information about current costs and utilization of nursing service personnel, more appropriate and cost-effective decisions can be made about assignment of nurses to various tasks.

EDUCATION

A knowledge base must be developed in management of human resources, organizational strategy, and information systems. Nurse managers must work to prepare their staff to understand the economics of health care and the cost impacts that nursing has on the entire health care delivery system. This education should encompass basic and advanced concepts in economics and financial management. We anticipate professional requirements for nurses will include being knowlegeable about the new payment system. Because nursing is the largest component of the health professions, our understanding and acceptance of the case-mix system can do much to develop a positive philosophy that can encourage a productive attitude toward working in nursing.

The education for nursing must include an awareness of the vast role that computers and information processing will continue to play in management. Nursing will increasingly be identified as a business, and nurses will need to develop a more businesslike, managerial attitude toward practice. Because collaboration between nursing and other health care professionals will increase, the seminars and meetings educating them to the new changes in health care should be jointly arranged and attended.

Hospital structure is in the process of changing from a centralized to a decentralized organization, with a corporate type of administrative body. Organizational theory and the change process should be implicitly imparted to all nursing staff being educated to cope with the new legislatively mandated changes. It is anticipated that by the year 1995, multihospital systems will increase by 125 percent. Nurses should be educated for this corporate world.

Because of the nature of the new federal regulations monitoring the nature of case mix reviewed above, under the new system hospitals are continuing to regionalize and specialize. Nurses should be shown what specialties are being offered to the community and should be offered further opportunities for entering newly specialized roles. The clinical specialist role will become a model to emulate.

The new system emphasizes keeping patients out of the hospital, as well as striving to get them discharged as quickly as possible. Therefore, community health centers and long-term-care facilities will treat more complex cases and sicker patients. Further, there will be an increased demand for community nursing. Nurses should be urged on the undergraduate, graduate, and professional levels to concern themselves with a changing hospital, and the resulting community nursing, case mix. In addition, the preventative or wellness promotion component to health care must be increased to keep patients out of the hospitals while keeping nursing at the forefront of the health care professions.

As mentioned above, because much of the management decision-making process depends on perceptions of personnel performance, there is a great need for nursing to market itself. We must examine the services that nursing offers to determine whether those services are what the consumer really wants or needs. The first step would be to conduct an environmental and community assessment. Professional education efforts should include offerings on marketing principles.

RESEARCH

An area of deficiency in nursing has been research in the clinical setting. The transition from measuring the hospital product from hospital descriptors to patient diagnosis-related descriptors will make nursing research more identifiable or case-oriented. In this way the research will be more meaningful to the nursing community, which is accustomed to clinical analysis. As the budgetary cutbacks continue, the cost justification for nursing research must continually be reinforced.

Research needs to be directed toward assisting with documentation that *nursing makes a difference.* The kinds of issues that must be stressed include what nursing has done to reduce length of stay, the increasingly developed base of nursing in clinical documentation offered by the new system, and the need for correlating case mix and nursing diagnoses. Even under situations offering scanty resources, these types of cost-saving research measures might well be supported. Further, research concerning quality assurance, overall patient education and planning for the patient's discharge, and preparation for the patient's discharge in order to reduce patient return to hospital, would meet the kinds of research standards demanded. Utilization review occurs within 24 hours of admission and is carried out by the UR coordinator, who reviews the patient's medical record, ascertains the tentative diagnosis, and determines the approximate length of stay. Nurses must then incorporate this information on tentative diagnosis and expected length of stay into their discharge planning for the patient.

Nursing should be very much aware of outliers in the same terms that the federal government is using to computerize its monitoring system for detecting excess in this area. The government is increasingly demanding justification for outlier status and its review explores whether patients are "cost" or "length-of-stay" outliers. Nursing has to be aware that resource use is exaggerated in outlier cases. By reviewing the management information reports, nursing should be able to spot the principal diagnoses where outliers tend to occur.

Case mix, by definition, encourages nursing research in the clinical setting. It permits interhospital comparisons by the very nature of the management information reports. This could develop multi-institutional collaboration on research in projects that would thereby develop economies of scale for cost-effectiveness. All individual hospitals involved would benefit enormously.

Research needs to be conducted on case mix and the model of the delivery of nursing services. Specifically, the need for primary care and support services needs to be researched and compared with the cost-effectiveness of team nursing with skill-level fragmentation.

The community provision of nursing services must be researched because the cost of these services is currently lower than the same services offered to inpatients. With the case-mix system proliferating and reducing the number of inpatients, measures should be taken to make certain that the same cost levels are maintained in the community to ensure that nurses are properly compensated for their rendering of quality care. In short, we want community care to remain less expensive (minimal overhead costs) while maintaining appropriately competitive staff salaries. By controlling the escalation of overhead, community care services can remain less expensive than hospital services while appropriately competitive staff salaries are maintained.

CONCLUSION

Nursing, with increased effort and awareness, can become the leading edge of the federal government's newly instituted cost reduction measures. If education, human resource development, organization skills, and information managemnt techniques are developed and maintained in tandem with the newly instituted changes in Medicare reimbursement outlined above, the future for nursing could well spell unlimited expansion of its health care and its management responsibility.

NURSING GEARS UP
FOR DRGs:
MANAGEMENT STRATEGIES
Franklin A. Shaffer

The organizational changes that are gradually falling into place as a result of the new prospective payment system most prominently include participative management and decentralization. What specific indicators can provide us with a better understanding of these organizational trends?

First, top management has traditionally perceived the hospital as divided into the distinct departments of medical staff, administration, finance, nursing, and laboratory. Under the new system, however, a new department, actually in existence before but previously understood as part of the financial department, emerges in its own right. This is the *medical records department.*

Of importance is that the new system merges clinical and financial data in the same computerized system and in the same management information reports. This never happened under the old system, which organized the financial data separately from the clinical data, and where the medical and the financial information systems operated as two autonomous spheres of influence connected only by limited communication at the time of discharge and billing.

Under the new prospective payment system, by its very name "prospective," we can see at once that payment—or billing—is formulated *before* the patient is even admitted. A price exists for 467 possible diagnostic categories, which will cover the vast majority of the patients admitted to the hospital. So the record of the *admission* rather than the record of the *treatment* now governs payment to the hospital for the patient's care, which has serious implications for the hospital's solvency because costs over the amount that the federal government determines to be appropriate for each diagnosis will come out of the hospital's profits. This has resulted in a fusing of the two previously autonomous hospital functions, treatment and billing, in the medical record. This merger is emblematic of increased communication between the various departments in the hospital, a result of the mandatory prospective payment system.

So top hospital management must respond to the changes, and because the record of the clinical diagnosis spells a specific dollar amount for the hospital's cash register, the status of the *medical record* of the clinical diagnosis has been elevated. The classification and coding of patient conditions according to 467 categories will be monitored by the federal government. What are some of the specific transitional responses that we are beginning to see in the top-level management of hospitals across the country?

EXECUTIVE MANAGEMENT'S ROLE

Information Systems

Because the hallmark of prospective payment is the merging of clinical and financial data by DRG (diagnosis related group), new information systems are the first component discussed by top management as part of the transition. The new information, combining patient and operational data, will be used throughout the hospital for management purposes other than payment. These purposes include financial monitoring, utilization management, marketing, and product planning. New channels will be created for sharing and presenting data to departments within the institution.

Computer literacy. Different kinds of reports will be required for management personnel in different positions—data alone are meaningless unless they are organized and presented logically. The key to accomplishing this indispensable function is a sophisticated information system. Indeed, only the reduction of time between data collection and data retrieval through *computers* has made the DRG system possible in the first place.

So, in a sense the computer revolution is the historical spawning ground that has brought the prospective payment system into existence, and in many ways the learning process involved in becoming *computer literate* parallels the learning process involved in becoming familiar with and expert at using the new prospective payment system. Computer reports—the fruit of an information management system—intimidate many people in organizations undergoing management transitions in the same way that computers have traditionally been used to intimidate everyone from the top to the bottom of the society at large.

Management personnel have understood that getting information and hands-on contact with reports, files, records, data, facts, and statistics is power. Now, these sources of power are changing, and this is causing an enormous increase in anxiety. Well that it should, because power relationships are entirely rearranged by the new technology. But the coping strategies required to contain and alleviate this anxiety and to turn it to productive ends require a quiet insistence that *all* personnel learn to read the appropriate computerized reports. This is not possible without two prerequisites: an effective information management system and a mechanism for providing the information to those managers who are highly motivated. These prerequisites explain we began by addressing top management. This is the level at which decisions are made and power exists to purchase the sophisticated computer technology required to properly manage a large organization.

QUALITY ASSURANCE

The *raison d'etre* or, in the terminology of the prospective payment system, the *product* of the hospital is patient care. This is what the institution sells and is the commodity for which it is reimbursed. It is hoped that a hospital will not sacrifice the quality of its care in order to become more efficient. The first task of management, then, is to implement strategies geared to assuring that the changes encouraged by the DRG system do not reduce the quality of the care offered.

Under the new system, clinical departments will receive such data as physician performance profiles. These data were never available before. They place physicians under public scrutiny to an extent never before imagined. How will clinical personnel react to these data? Some doctors will be seen—in the eyes of the hospital—as more efficient at treating cases that bring in more revenue. The hospital's attitude toward particular physicians will be governed by new elements entirely, particularly in relation to efficiency criteria.

Whether these new criteria will be viewed as destructive or constructive will depend upon whether management presents them as "treatment shortcuts" or "reallocation of expensive resources to areas of greatest need." The former approach fosters ineffective management, while the latter policy encourages the medical staff as a whole to expend time and resources on those areas of the hospital product—direct and indirect patient care—that most require care. In this context, it is now possible to see why management strategy is so vital to the success or failure of the implementation of the new system.

The perspective of the physicians involved requires quality assurance that will be considered invalid without the appropriate presentation of the system as a care enhancer rather than a care reducer. It is hoped that patients *who really need care* will receive care, and that patients *who really do not need care* will not be permitted to absorb costly resources that could be better allocated. This is not 1950; resources are now limited, and new management strategies require conservation and careful allocation. Physicians who continue to overutilize resources will find hospitals reluctant to grant them staff privileges. We are entering an era of difficult ethical/moral decision making due to limited resources.

MANAGEMENT STRUCTURE

The most important challenge to top hospital management, as mentioned, will be to encourage interdepartmental and multidisciplinary communication to identify potential areas for cost savings and increased efficiency. This must involve the creation of an organizational climate that rewards efficiency, beginning with programs demanding that employees learn to read computer reports.

PROSPECTIVE PRICING COMMITTEE

That the changes involved with prospective pricing are sweeping has been emphasized again and again. *How* sweeping, however, cannot be absorbed by a given readership or a given audience until the discussion falls upon the institution of a prospective pricing committee that is formed by hospital management to involve staff in the transition. The changes could continue unnoticed until this gesture influences the hospital's management in a visible way. Therefore, to expedite the process of transition, to show that the organization is serious about a change in management, one of the first organizational changes should be appointing an interdisciplinary prospective pricing committee composed of persons from executive management, medical staff, and middle management. Generally, hospital management is represented according to defined institutional structures, which usually include the areas of finance, patient billing, medical records, nursing, data processing, and management engineering. A major outcome of the prospective pricing committee is as a vehicle of "team-building."

COMMITTEE CHAIRPERSON

A member of the executive management team chairs the prospective payment committee. The person chosen must be respected, action-oriented, and known to be a forceful, vital member of the hospital executive staff with excellent communications skills. Without this kind of visible authority, making the prospective payment committee a respected institution can become difficult. Inertia is generally the hallmark in bureaucracies, particularly hospitals, where patient intake and processing continues relentlessly, without regard for institutional infrastructure enhancements.

UTILIZATION MANAGEMENT

Concurrent review of the hospital product's management should replace the retrospective review that has historically neglected to monitor waste and inefficiency *as they took place*. The advantage of the new system is that information dissemination concerning hospital product (that is, direct and indirect patient care) affords day-to-day feedback concerning price overruns for particular diagnoses. The presumption behind the system is that, if other hospitals can manage a particular diagnosis for less money, then the hospital presently managing the same diagnosis should also be able to manage for less. The burden of proof for inefficiency thus transfers to the individual hospital.

HUMAN RESOURCES MANAGEMENT

Nursing immediately comes to mind when this category of the hospital product is mentioned, since nursing is labor-intensive. The new system seeks to reduce unproductive labor hours. As mentioned above, the system's information system should permit the matching of case mix with appropriate manpower. This should take acuteness of the patient's condition and volume of services into consideration. These principles, also reviewed above, should be applied to supplies and inventory management.

MEDICAL STAFF

Frequently, physicians resist cost-consciousness in the name of quality assurance. This has been discussed repeatedly and will again be repeated; physicians must be educated to the fact that resources for quality assurance are no longer unlimited. It is now a situation of maximizing limited resources rather than one of allocating unlimited resources. The *relative* condition of the patient is the issue, not the *absolute* condition. That is, one patient's receiving treatment may well deprive another of treatment that is even more urgently needed. Understanding the interplay between computer-generated cost data and the entire case mix in the hospital—the patients being treated by other physicians—can help to optimally allocate scarce hospital resources among a more-accurately understood case mix. Physicians must come to see themselves more as a team servicing the same population rather than as individuals isolated from the rest of the hospital staff. Across the U.S., physicians are becoming involved with the DRG payment system. The prospective payment system does not dictate medical practice; it states the rate for DRGs.

EDUCATION

The committee operates as an interface between the technical information generally available concerning the DRG system and the unique needs of the particular hospitals newly entered into the system. Generally, the members of the committee themselves do not understand all there is to know about DRGs, and their self-education is crucial to their being able to fullfill their function of educating the rest of the hospital community. To accomplish this function, the committee must disseminate its members throughout the institution, allocating its manpower multidimensionally in order to set the precedents and channels of communication that later will come to be conduits for information.

This educational stage can also serve to test the hospital's management channels for receptivity and positive attitudinal development concerning the new system. Because the information's dissemination and the hierarchy's decentralization requires computer literacy development and facility with report reading at all levels, incentives for this kind of orientation should be part of the educational strategy.

MEDICAL RECORDS

Errors in coding patients' diagnoses according to the DRG system constitute one of the more difficult problems in the system's implementation. To rectify this pitfall, as in other problem areas of the system, not only the medical records department, but all staff responsible for documenting the patients' records must be involved. The accurate completion and coding of the medical record and the patient's bill are paramount for the success of the DRG system and for the continued solvency of the hospital under the new federal monitoring constraints.

INFORMATION SYSTEMS

It is not only the raw price/diagnosis data that the DRG system is capable of generating. The managerial implications of these data, when manipulated and stored in a manner useful for product-oriented reports, are far-reaching, providing that the proper reports are circulated effectively throughout the hospital. Operational and productivity information is calculated by many computer-based systems on the basis of the hospital's case mix. This permits more efficient management of the hospital product by proper staffing and scheduling according to the kinds of patient needs discernible from the case-mix data. Nursing staffing and scheduling, and equipment and supplies management, are particularly responsive to proper information generation from price/diagnosis data for any given hospital.

ANTICIPATED CHANGES IN ORGANIZATIONAL STRUCTURE

Medical records' increased importance may require extensive integration with the functions served by finance, patient billing, and utilization management. The prospective payment committee must act to supervise this organizational transition. The personnel may require reallocation or interdepartmental reassignment to integrate clinical/payment functions, heretofore separately maintained.

DRG COORDINATOR'S ROLE

Some hospitals may find it expeditious to supplement the efforts of the prospective payment committee with the appointment of a DRG coordinator. Others may find that this figure vitiates the absorption of the new system's impact and slows the adaptation process by confining the DRG effort too securely in one individual. The important idea here, as in other areas of implementation, is that the transition in information management and departmental reorganization and decentralization must be made according to the unique needs and capabilities of every hospital. This is a time of testing each institution's vitality. Whatever means are necessary to maintain institutional product quality while increasing efficiency must be adopted.

SOME SPECIFIC MEASURES FOR TOP MANAGEMENT

The transitional period will look something like the sample scenario presented here. First, the DRG case-mix cost-reporting system will be established. The true cost of hospital services will be ascertained by establishing cost accounting systems. The services in the hospital product that compare *favorably* with the DRG pricing will be called "winners" or producers of hospital profit, and the services in the hospital product that compare *unfavorably* with the DRG pricing will be called "losers," or producers of hospital losses. HCFA provides a grouping program that can be used to determine DRG assignment prior to billing. This will be acquired and established in the billing system as part of patient intake. Medical chart documentation and processing will be expedited by better training of coders and enforcing suspension of privileges.

The prospective payment committee, authoritatively backed and energetically supervised by the CEO of the hospital, as well as by prominent physicians, will be responsible for monitoring hospital personnel awareness of the implementation of the new system. This will include supervision of increased ancillary service capabilities to support physician practice through more timely reporting of test results and weekend coverage. Downward skill substitution will thus be mitigated as highly paid staff members will be able to attend to their appropriate functions. Nursing, as will be seen in the section below concerning that hospital department, will also benefit enormously from the implementation of these cost-saving measures.

Discharge planning will be improved by the observance of a new system of regulations governing pre-admission screening, on-admission testing, and patient education. The length of stay for the patient will be understood at the time of admission, psychologically predisposing patient, staff, and physician to predefine parameters governing the quality of hospital product allocated for treatment. Underlying all of these preparations, of course, will be a continual awareness of what the hospital will be reimbursed for the patient's diagnosis under the prospective payment system.

Physician feedback will be obtained concerning the appropriateness of the length of stay as set forth by the DRG categories. Quality assurance will incorporate this feedback. A vital part of the new system is the implementation of a mandatory procedure requiring that the physicians review patient bills as part of grand rounds. The time consumed in this effort, if top management has fulfilled its primary responsibility of effective information dissemination by computer or whatever equipment is necessary, will be practically nothing.

Patient DRGs that are "profitable" will be encouraged more than DRGs that are not. The treatment of these patients will be marketed by the hospital, and physicians and other medical staff predisposed to treat such cases should be given corresponding incentives. Here again, ethics will become a major issue: who cares for the "losers"?

Department budget and expense account procedures will be controlled by the new management accountability structure using productivity measures calculated according to the DRG assignment and case-mix definition. Staffing will be monitored according to productive and nonproductive paid hours, which will be quickly calculated on the basis of case mix treated according to the accuracy and timeliness of the new information-management reports.

Exchange carts will be employed on patient units and in operating rooms to reduce the costs of medical and surgical supplies ordinarily wasted during the normal operation of the previous retrospective billing procedures.

Sophisticated financial analysis capabilities will be implemented that will perment study and correction of high-cost management areas. Clinical services and clinical departments, DRG coordination, medical records, utilization review, patient billing, and discharge planning will be monitored continuously to assure effective and efficient operations. The organizational structures must be modified and maintained to ensure higher levels of physician and management accountability for continuous measurement of financial impact of their management decisions.

Mangement will prepare and be ready to deliver its rationale underlining the importance of staff reductions, cost monitoring, and the development of ancillary services as means of ensuring the hospital's viability in an enconomically contracted environment while maintaining quality.

This rationale will be presented in order to counter both community concern with quality and employee opposition to staff reductions.

THE NURSING DEPARTMENT

To understand the implications of the management strategies outlined above for the nursing department, the importance of top management's information dissemination function cannot be overstated. The decentralization of the hospital's cost-monitoring system from the financial office to the various departments depends on top management's dissemination of management information reports tailored to the individual hospital's needs and, moreover, to the individual department's needs.

The hospital must conduct human resources management seminars designed to invest its nursing department personnel with an understanding of computer literacy. More important, however, is an aggressive attitude on the part of the nurse executive in the hospital toward acquiring these management skills and in taking an active role in the transition.

Nursing, because of its continuous contact with the patient community on a 24-hour basis, is the leading edge of quality assurance. If nursing can demonstrate that the hospital can provide increased quality services with a lower budget—because of:

- Reduced downward skill substitution,
- increased use of ancillary services,
- increased staffing efficiency according to accurate case mix reporting, and
- more accurate recording of clinical information and chart maintenance by professional nursing staff by timely updating data,

then nursing will, by definition, become the key ally for hospital management in its campaign to streamline costs and increase quality.

CHALLENGE TO THE NURSE EXECUTIVE

The first challenge to the nursing department will be the definition of essential nursing services and their maintenance and enhancement under reduced budgetary conditions. The managerial challenge to the nurse executive divides into three categories: fiscal, organizational, and communication. It should be emphasized here, however, that the nurse executive, as a person, must shoulder the managerial and developmental tasks of education in the economics of health care, the fiscal management of hospitals, the use of computers and information processing systems, and organizational dynamics and business administration. This attitude—incorporating an executive approach and a business orientation—must supplement clinical expertise in order to facilitate effective interaction with the financial department. The nurse executive might find it useful to employ a financial person to assist with the educational preparation of nurse managers and to secure their assistance in fiscal matters and to expedite working as a team member with the financial department.

FISCAL CHALLENGE

The effective contribution by nurse executives to the hospital's fiscal management presupposes their inclusion in the prospective payment committee membership, where they will work on an equal basis with the heads of other departments. The lack of reflection of nursing services as an autonomous entry in the hospital budget—nursing is still considered part of overhead—should not be similarly reflected in the prospective payment committee's allocation of responsibility to the nurse executive for fiscal management of nursing services. No one knows better what goes on in the nursing department.

The nurse executive should develop a patient classification system appropriate for the nursing case mix that parallels the medical classification system developed for the DRG system. This is a prerequisite of cost-effective, high-quality nursing. To accomplish this classification system so as to be able to appropriately allocate staffing, the application of a computerized management information system is necessary. Nursing-care costs should be determined according to patient diagnosis, age, intensity of nursing care required, and who provides the nursing care services.

Staffing must be monitored according to case mix as defined by the information management system designed and monitored in conjunction with the prospective payment committee. The staff profile in terms of salary, education, and experience must govern hiring of appropriate ancillary personnel to take up tasks inappropriately assumed by professional and experienced personnel. Professional staff may then be shifted to areas where their expertise is more essential.

Scheduling patterns must similarly follow the information generated by case mix. Concentration of too many personnel at the wrong time or in the wrong ward, according to the needs of the case mix, can produce both inefficient management and quality reduction. The data applied from a patient classification system can be employed on a departmental basis to justify budgetary requests at meetings of the hospital board or prospective payment committee.

The patient classification system employed must reflect the intensity of care needed and provided to patients so as to assure quality. It must predict the kinds of cases treated in the hospital. The characteristic potential in the hospital for overstaffing or understaffing must be identified. Once staffing problems are identified, a corrective action plan must be devised and implemented. The patient classification system is the first step in identifying nursing as a revenue-producing center.

By applying an effective patient classification system, the nurse abseteeism rate can be reduced by matching case-mix needs with appropriateness of staff education and scheduling.

As in many other areas of management, nursing department budgeting, staffing, and scheduling depend upon the accuracy and timeliness of the information generated in conjunction with the hospital management's computer system. It is up to the nurse executive to represent the nursing department's management information needs effectively and to disseminate the information designed to fill these needs on an ongoing basis. If the nurse executive fails to fulfill this function, the hospital will predictably be required, as part of the cost-cutting role that the government will require it to assume, to look elsewhere to fulfill it.

The nursing department must become responsible for educating the patient and his family at the time of admission concerning expected length of stay and discharge. This kind of cost-awareness behavior should be reinforced at all stages of the hospital stay. It must also be reinforced within the nursing department's day-to-day operation at the unit level. Indeed, individual members of the nursing staff providing patient care, must be able to understand computer reports in order to be able to monitor costs at the unit level.

This relates closely with the need for insistence, more than ever before, upon accurate documentation by the nursing staff. The stereotype of the nurse at the unit level who does not know where the chart is, or whether the patient has been given medication, or whether the appropriate dose has been given, must be eliminated by fail-safe protocols for monitoring documentation of care. Computers and other work-simplification techniques can be used to accomplish these tasks and to facilitate the accuracy of monitoring. Cost-consciousness concerning the allocation of supplies is also encouraged by the use of monitoring and recording techniques.

All of the above point to the importance of education programs within the nursing department that parallel or dovetail with the education programs instituted by the prospective payment committee. Seminars must be conducted to introduce key personnel to computer reports used for management information and case-mix monitoring.

ORGANIZATIONAL CHALLENGE

The inpatient care portion of the hospital product has traditionally been the nurse's domain. New products, however, are rapidly replacing a large portion of this part of the hospital product in the wake of cost-cutting measures inherent in the prospective payment system. Patients are leaving the hospital sicker, faster, and are entering less frequently and more reluctantly. In this context, community nursing services are being demanded on an increasing basis. Hospitals are rapidly diversifying by establishing a full range of services, including skilled nursing facilities and a myriad of home health services. Non-acute care in homes and centers is requested and offers expanded career options for nurses. If these are offered as part of hospital services—and it is the responsibility of the nurse executive to demand this option—the salary scale for nursing personnel providing this care can equal that for inpatient service.

As part of the new community offering, the hospital, and particularly the nurse executive, must take an active role in marketing the nursing department's image. If the nursing department is going to effectively expand the hospital's product into the community's homes to reserve hospital bed space for those patients who need it the most, then increased marketing of the nursing department as appropriately extended into the home must be effected. Identification and creation of nursing needs heretofore unaddressed—or allowed to diminish with time (such as house calls not requiring physicians) must be investigated, systematized, and marketed.

As can be seen in the definition of the nursing department's role in the prospective payment committee, the staff of the nursing department must be permitted to participate fully in hospital management interdepartmental, interdisciplinary, and decision-making activity.

COMMUNICATION CHALLENGE

Communication with nursing staff, medical staff, patient and family, and interdepartmental systems must be facilitated. As patients become selected or rejected by hospitals on the basis of the acuteness of their need for treatment, hospital length of stay will be shortened and hospital care intensified. Nursing staff will adopt increasingly greater responsibility for coordinating the care of patients. Communication systems are required for effectively fulfilling this responsibility of organizing the effort of the nursing staff, medical staff, and numerous other departments. Indeed, the nurse is the coordinator of care.

The nursing staff members are public relations personnel for the hospital to the community. The nursing department conveys the hospital's quality assurance commitment more than any other department. The impression conveyed depends largely on the organizational matters described above, including the effectiveness of information management strategies and the appropriateness of communication systems discussed here. Toward the end of effective communication, the nurse executive must establish it with the nursing staff, encouraging two-way interaction with ongoing staff feedback, staff education concerning the new system's institution, and clear and up-to-date delineation of the specific steps that the staff must take to implement the new payment plan.

Further, the nursing department must establish clear channels of communication with the medical staff including timely scheduling, completion, and evaluation of treatment procedures.

The nursing department also must communicate effectively with patients and their families to market the image of the nursing department and the hospital as a whole and to follow up on quality assurance by monitoring the response of the patients to the hospital product. This is nowhere more important than on the nursing unit itself, typically under the jurisdiction of the head nurse, and it is to the day-to-day changes in the operation of the nursing unit that will arise in response to the prospective payment system that we now turn.

THE NURSING UNIT

The nursing unit providing the direct patient care is the front line of the hospital operation. Paramount in the effort made in this article to introduce the changes that must accompany the new propsective payment plan is the understanding that all of the management planning, strategy, computer power, expertise, and manpower training are useless unless they are accompanied by effective strategies for implementation at the unit level.

The preceding discussion focused primarily on the administrative portion of the maintenance and assurance of the quality of the hospital product more than on the actual treatment portion traditionally reserved for the nursing unit. The head nurse will be the focus of this discussion, because this individual is the interface between the nursing department and the reforms experienced there and between the overall hospital management and the reforms experienced there as a result of instituting the prospective payment system.

How will day-to-day changes unfold on the front lines in the hospital—on the nursing unit—after the transition has been made to prospective payment? There are three fundamental areas in which the head nurse will become proficient that will alter the present configuration of management on the nursing unit. These are information management skills, staffing skills emanating from improved information management skills, and allocation of the nursing function more efficiently by using ancillary personnel to adopt tasks misapplying labor power in examples of cross-subsidization and downward skills substitution.

Allocation of supplies will be streamlined according to case mix, and communication with the nurse executive will function on a level more informed by intelligent interpretation of computer reports and monitoring of documentation procedures of patient care. Quality assurance will be increased by improved computer or other work-simplification systems designed to streamline documentation of care. Early prognosis and documenting of complications will, therefore, be possible.

Departmental meetings and seminars conducted by the nurse executive would be attended by the head nurses to learn proper application of information management to staffing, supply ordering, scheduling, and maintaining documentation. These meetings would parallel those conducted on a hospital-wide basis for top management and would involve intensive feedback from personnel so as to maintain morale. This is extremely important to emphasize in the context of a high probability of nursing staff cutbacks. The need for understanding the operation of the prospective payment system and the cost-reduction effort that it represents toward efficiently applying reduced resources to the patients who need them the most should help maintain morale at the unit level. Education concerning the opportunities within the community itself outside of the hospital (for instance, in homes) is fundamental to maintaining morale.

Accountability systems must be implemented at the unit level, with increased responsibility vested in the head nurse as sophistication with information management report interpretation grows. The attitude of the head nurse toward the medical record of the patient must become integrated with the entire hospital's changed view of this record. Cost must be interpreted in relation to everything that happens on the ward, and the head nurse must be held accountable for cost variations in treatment of patients whose care exceeds the levels established by the appropriate DRG. The nursing staff needs to know the hospital's marketing initiatives. They should have access to data that identify the ''losers''and the ''winners'' on their specific unit, and they should incorporate this information into the nursing department's short- and long- range planning. Similarly, staffing and scheduling on the wards must be accomplished in view of the case mix and the needs of the patients who occupy the beds— not in view of the formerly uninformed guess of the staffing personnel.

Supplies must be ordered in view of the case mix, as well; again, it is clear that the design of the nursing department's information management reports by the nurse executive is fundamental to their proper interpretation and use by the head nurse. But, conversely, the head nurse must be held accountable for feedback concerning the timeliness, accuracy, and usefulness of the manipulation and presentation of the data on these reports. As such, the nurse executive must *listen* to the head nurse—as mentioned above, communication must be regular and ongoing and *two-way*. Otherwise, the ward will operate inefficiently, outside of the mainstream of the hospital's best organizational effort.

SUMMARY

In summary, nursing, in gearing up for DRGs, needs to identify and/or use the following:

- The nursing case mix profile;

- the staff mix needed to care for the case mix;

- standards of nursing practice for case mix;

- nonnursing activities performed by staff nurses themselves (cross-subsidization and downward skill subsitituion.

- management reports to invoke cost consciousness on the part of nursing staff;

- quality assurance audits to correlate length of stay with nursing costs; and
- the correlation of nursing productivity and case mix.

The magnitude of the importance of computer technology and computer literacy has been emphasized. The need to warn of the impending transformation of health care has been replaced in the discussion presented here by a presupposition that specific strategies must be developed. The focus has shifted from the theoretical to the tactical and, while this is by no means a signal for complacency, it is nonetheless a step in the right direction, particularly for nursing.

DRGs: IMPERATIVE STRATEGIES FOR NURSING SERVICE ADMINISTRATION

Rosalinda M. Toth

Although the majority of health and illness care in the United States is provided by nurses, physicians and hospital bureaucrats have maintained the control over who receives care, the type of care received, and by whom it is rendered. It has long been assumed by those in control that nursing is a branch of medicine. It is not! It must be autonomous if it is to survive as a profession, and herein lies the dilemma.

As Kohnke so aptly stated,

> Nursing is dedicated to the care of illness, but its large concern is with the health care of society. It strives for the development of maximum health potential of all social groups by predicting or diagnosing the potential or actual health problems as well as delivering the care necessary to heal and rehabilitate the sick and disabled. To assist man in reaching his maximum health potential, the profession must possess a substantial body of knowledge and a professional nursing group capable of using this knowledge in the service of society. . . . In developing from a semiprofessional group to a professional group, [nursing] has gained this knowledge and has also gained the professionals capable of using it. Therefore, nursing has the ability to maintain the autonomy of full professional status.[1]

But what authority have we exercised over the problem of rising health care costs or its possible resolution?

It is a simple fact of life that money is power: the power to control, to bargain, to exploit, to create change, to design and implement new ideas, and the power to achieve self-actualization.

Aristotle once said that money is ''a guarantee that we may have what we

---

[1]M. Kohnke, *The Case for Consultation in Nursing* (New York: John Wiley and Sons, 1978), p. 1-2.

want in the future. Tho we need nothing at the moment, it ensures the possibility of satisfying a necessary desire when it arises.''[2]

Not one of us in nursing today denies the tremendous power that physicians exert in the hospital industry, because physicians supply that industry with dollars through their admission practices.

It is also a fact that departments of nursing are the largest spenders of health care dollars in hospitals. These departments are labor-intensive and historically have not been held accountable for their services monetarily.

There are several reasons for this. Until recently, directors of nursing were excellent bedside practitioners who, through longevity, worked their way up the corporate ladder. Credentialing was considered unimportant, and sound business practices were not expected. Secondly, most directors of nursing were women in a male-dominated hierarchy, and nurses, by virtue of their history, are viewed by the health care bureaucracy as powerless. They are predominantly white, middle-class females whom society has taught to be submissive, docile, and pleased to be governed by men.[3] Thirdly, and closely allied, is the obvious (and enormous amount of) exploitive power to maintain the status quo of the hierarchy itself.

Since the first premise is rapidly changing, with more and more directors of nursing required to meet certain educational criteria, and with the profession itself promulgating education that includes business management skills, I'd like to expand upon the last premise—exploitation—especially as it relates to sexual bias.

Exploitation of Nurses

Exploitive power, according to May, is the simplest and most destructive kind of power. It is subjecting persons to whatever use they may have to the one who holds power.[4] Slavery, for example, is a form of exploitation. May continues, "This kind of power is exercised by those who have been radically rejected, whose lives are so barren that they know no way of relating to other people, except exploitation. It is even sometimes rationalized as the 'masculine' way of dealing with women.''[5]

Exploitation connotes force; wanted actions are rewarded, unwanted actions punished, by the exploiter. During the process, no input is required of the exploited person other than that he or she obey. No intelligence is necessary and, in fact, thinking, problem solving, and creativity are strongly discouraged. The result is total control by the exploiter.

Let me equate this to the current health care delivery system. Until recently, nursing service directors had very little control over their practice in hospitals.

---

[2]E. Brussell, Ed., *Dictionary of Quotable Definitions* (Englewood Cliffs, NJ: Prentice Hall, Inc., 1970), p. 379.

[3]J. M. Player, "The Economic Importance of Nurses," *Nursing Management,* 13(11):52, November 1982.

[4]R. May, *Power and Innocence* (New York: Dell Publishing Company, 1972), p. 105.

[5]*Ibid.*

Standards of care were set by bureaucrats and nurses under physician-dominated state agencies. Implementation of care was controlled by hospital administrators whose primary concern was the budget. Methods of care were controlled by physician-dominated boards or groups. The nurse simply did as she was directed through policy and procedures that she had no part in designing and was paid by a system that saw her as an assistant to the physician and therefore worth a secondary salary.

Unfortunately, many nurses and others associated with nursing hold onto these old ways and old ideas. They believe that it is the nurses' function to help physicians. They belittle education and do not want authority because it assumes personal responsibility. They believe that closer identification with another profession such as medicine will provide them with more prestige, and they accept without question a work structure that is indicative of a parent-child relationship where knowledge, wisdom, and rewards are doled out at the knee to "good girls and boys."

Nursing is about to reach adulthood, and we can no longer hang onto these old trappings. Likewise, hospital care has become big business. Different needs are felt, and a higher level of sophistication is required to operate efficiently.

The DRG system in New Jersey has had some responsibility for forcing these changes, thereby helping to create the dilemma that I mentioned earlier. The question at hand is: Do we maintain the older, paternal, exploitive structure, or does nursing become a true partner in the delivery of health care in New Jersey hospitals? Who makes this choice? As a nurse and hospital administrator, it seems logical that I am in the best position to choose, because I have the expertise (and the ability, therefore) to account for my services. However, I also recognize that I cannot make the decision or even be a part of this choice unless I also gain the management expertise necessary to operate within the DRG structure.

If this sounds rebellious, it is. However, as May states,

> The rebel is necessary as the lifeblood of culture, as the very root of civilization . . . the rebel is . . . one who breaks with established custom or tradition . . . He seeks above all an internal change, a change in the attitudes, emotions, and outlook of the people to whom he is devoted . . . Every act of rebellion tacitly presupposes some value. The rebel is the one who realizes that the master is as much imprisoned, if not as painfully, as he is by the institution of slavery; he rebels against that system which permits slaves and masters. His rebellion, if successful, saves the master also from the indignity of owning slaves.[6]

Today, nursing is rebelling. We need only look at statistics for verification. All over this country, nurses are unionizing, an overt demonstration of their dissatisfaction with the status quo, with empty promises, and with scapegoating tactics.

And no other labor force is experiencing the massive exits from that force as is nursing. If this exodus occurred in any other area, especially one that is male-dominated, there would be a universal, human outcry that the system

---

[6]*Ibid.* p. 220-222.

that employs them is an unmitigated disaster. But where is the outcry for nursing? Instead, new ways are promulgated that simply manipulate the old structure, dress it up, tie it with a bow, but essentially change nothing and perpetuate the master-slave concept. Worse yet is the fact that the current masters do not even ask the slaves what they want. Instead, the slaves are told what they want and what they need to make them happy slaves.

Is it really any wonder that, probably for the first time in our history, organized nursing has chosen to defy the medical profession and the hospital association to support fully a financial system such as DRG? And, to make matters worse, in New Jersey at least, to have had the audacity to demand input on the design of the system and to fight for that area (namely RIMs) that allows us to calculate in cold dollars and cents our value to the health care delivery system?

And that brings me to purpose of this article. DRGs are imperative for efficient nursing management, and RIMs are an invaluable tool that must not be allowed to be rejected by a system that fears our autonomy.

Efficient Nursing Management

It is time to begin internalizing the fee-for-service concept for nursing in hospitals. Generally, the very mention of this idea causes sweaty palms, cold feet, and shivering spines on the part of some hospital administrators. For it is viewed as a preemption to individual contracting and independent practice, and as a potential increase in collective bargaining units, all of which connote loss of power or, at best, loss of centralized power.

However, progressive administrators see it for what it really is: a method of accurately defining nursing care in terms of money. The fee-for-service concept simply provides a method for identifying *quantitatively* the variations in nursing care rendered to hospitalized patients based on their nursing care needs. A true cost-accounting system for services rendered strengthens the overall financial structure of an institution and provides the basis for efficient and effective management principles.

I don't think that anyone today would argue that using a per diem rate for nursing care is an adequate measure for consumption of services. Nursing care cannot be apportioned equally each and every day for each and every patient because patient needs change each and every day for each and every patient. Even the New Jersey State Department of Health recognized that "a per diem rate for an illness condition implies that each and every patient with the same affliction will display identical use of nursing services . . . this approach is insensitive to the varying amount of nursing time consumed by patients . . . ."[7] It is the antithesis of the fee-for-service concept.

RIMs, on the other hand, are "a measure of resource use derived from nursing activity . . . used to distribute reported general nursing costs based upon

---

[7]New Jersey State Department of Health. *A Prospective Reimbursement System Based on Patient Case-Mix for New Jersey Hospitals: Case-Mix Reimbursement and DRG Nursing-Cost Allocation,* 1976-1983, p. 4.

the relationship between nursing activity and nursing costs. A RIM, which is based on the actual delivery of nursing service to patients, therefore represents a more functional allocation unit than does the use of the patient day'': ergo, fee for service.[8]

How do we use this system both for nursing and, more importantly, for the structure itself (for to strengthen one is to strengthen the other)? Remember, the United States became strong and great as a democracy, which included the eventual abolition of slavery. So, too, with health care.

The Nursing Management Report

The most useful tool for nursing managers operating within DRGs is the management report. Generally, these are sent to fiscal officers. Directors of nursing service must also receive a copy. Make appropriate arrangements with your fiscal officer to get a copy when it arrives at your institution. Do not be thwarted by comments that you don't need it or, worse yet, that it is useless without his (the fiscal officer's) interpretation.

Figure 1 is a prototype nursing management report. Column 1 identifies the DRG by number, with the English descriptor alongside in column 2. It would also be helpful to have a personal copy of the DRG list regulation. Request one from your administrator or write to the New Jersey State Department of Health and request the newest one, dated January 7, 1982. This describes each of the 467 DRGs and their 23 MDCs, gives the outlier trim points for each DRG, and identifies clinical outlier DRGs.

Column 3 of the management report indicates the number of cases of each DRG that you had in your hospital. This is extremely important. You want to be aware of patterns and trends. What are the predominant DRGs that you treat? Can you equate rises and falls in certain DRGs by season? These data can tell you what kind of nursing expertise you need. For example, you don't need a diabetic clinician if you only treat 100 diabetics a year, but you may need an enterostomal therapist if you see 400 ostomies a year. If you have a sharp increase in coronaries in winter but relatively few the rest of the year, perhaps you would do better to contract with a cardiac clinician full time for four months during the winter rather than paying a full-time yearly salary for someone who may well be underutilized during the summer months. If it's a high-volume DRG that you are looking at, do you have a specialized unit for consolidation of resources?

You will also need these data for comparative analyses. For example, last year you only treated 12 fractured hips, but this year, in the first six months, you already treated 54. What does this mean? Has your staff received the necessary continuing education to handle these patients? Will you have to reevaluate the utilization of your orthopedic operating room? Who sets up and maintains traction apparatus? What kind of relationship will there have to be with the physical therapy department for the rehabilitation phases? Using these

---
[8]*Ibid.*

Figure 1. Prototype nursing management report.

DRG	Description	Number of Cases	Hospital Rank	State Rank	Average Length of Stay	Total Nursing Cost (All Pts.)	Average Nursing Cost Per Case	Percent Nursing Cost of DRG	Nursing Rank All DRGs
039	Lens O.R. Procedure	310	6	9	3.34H 3.25S	37,897.H 34,747.S	122.25H 112.09S	24.69	15
243	Back Disorder Medical	208	21	21	8.50H 8.75S	76,641.H 65,099.S	368.47H 312.98S	49.09	1
122	Circulatory Disorder with AMI, D/C Alive without cardiovascular complications Medical	144	10	14	13.13H 14.67S	199,943.H 208,224.S	1,388.00H 1,446.00S	78.63	2
441	Hand Procedure for injury	6	252	219	1.50H 2.20S	729.H 966.S	122.00H 161.00S	33.47	253
177	Ulcer without complications Age 70 +, Medical	14	157	145	9.43H 8.85S	10,640.H 7,686.S	760.00H 549.00S	64.80	104
202	Cirrhosis and/or Alcoholic hepatitis	23	97	114	12.13H 11.00S	20,360.H 16,652.S	885.00H 605.00S	63.98	50

data, you can plan services before they are needed instead of waiting until a crisis arises.

Column 4 indicates how this particular DRG rates within your facility. For example, on this prototype report, the sixth-most-seen patient is in DRG 039. The least-admitted DRG is 441, which ranks 252nd. This assists you in quickly identifying the predominant conditions in your institution and helps in determining the resources necessary to efficiently handle these patients.

Column 5 describes where you fall with each DRG in comparison with all other hospitals. Although DRG 039 is your highest reading, sixth, it only rates ninth for the rest of the state. In other words, you treat a relatively higher number of cataract patients than most other hospitals.

Column number 6 indictes the average length of stay for each DRG. This is probably the single most important statistic on this report, for reimbursement by DRG rate depends upon length of stay. On the management report, there are two figures; one labeled H for hospital, one labeled S for state. The average length of stay for DRG 039 in this hospital is 3.34 days, compared to 3.25 days for all other hospitals in the state, so you know that you keep your cataract patients in the hospital slightly longer than other hospitals.

Length of stay is the major area in which nurses can have an impact on the entire reimbursement system. Physicians control the admission of patients, but registered nurses can, if they choose, control the dollar by controlling the discharge of these patients. This can be done through several different methods. By becoming familiar with each DRG's standard length of stay, the sharp unit manager (such as the head nurse) might remind a physician that a patient is coming close to the standard length of stay. Has discharge planning begun? Is the patient ready to go home? Does the patient need more intensive care provided by the nursing staff to make sure that the patient is discharged within that length of stay? Likewise, the nurse may advise the physician that the patient is nearing the length-of-stay standard but that, in the nurse's judgment, he is not ready for discharge. She may recommend to the physician why the patient needs to be kept an extra day or so—for example, for nursing teaching. If joint care plans are established in your institution (that is, care plans established by physician and nurse together as colleagues beginning on the day of admission), there is no reason why the care cannot be planned within the length-of-stay standard so that you can predict when the patient will be ready for discharge from the very first day of admission.

Column 7 indicates the total nursing cost incurred by all patients within that DRG in that hospital. On this report, you can see that a fairly costly DRG is 243, back disorders. You treat a relatively high number of cases, 208, but no higher than other hospitals, since you rate 21, as does the state average. Why, then, is the DRG 243 so costly? Your length of stay is below the state standard, so you are not keeping patients too long, thereby incurring cost that way.

In column 8, we see two figures again. The average nursing cost per case in this DRG in your hospital is indicated by the H, and the average nursing cost per case in this DRG in all other hospitals is indicated by the S. In DRG 243, we see that the nursing cost per case in this hospital is much higher than the state average.

Column 9 indicates the nursing cost percentage of each DRG. This represents the percentage of total nursing cost of the total DRG cost; in DRG 039, nursing represents 24.69 percent of the total cost. DRG 122 represents the highest nursing percentage, with nursing representing 78.63 percent of the total cost.

The last column indicates how each DRG rates in this institution with regard to nursing cost; DRG 243 ranks first, or is the highest-costing DRG for nursing.

So what does this tell us? We can immediately identify the most costly DRG, 243. We don't see any more than other hospitals, so chances are that we aren't doing anything significantly different from other hospitals or we'd be receiving more referrals. Our length of stay is lower than the state average. So what's wrong?

The management report is not designed to solve our problems, merely to help us identify them. Armed with these data, I now know that, as director of the nursing service, I have to focus on nursing management of these patients to find out what is happening.

There are certain assumptions that I can make at the outset that will help me focus in on where and how to study the problem. If this report were for my institution, I would know, for example, that:

1. All DRG 243 patients are admitted to my orthopedic unit. Therefore, I can assume that the nurses on this unit are familiar enough with this problem and that they know how to manage patient care effectively. This is further substantiated by this DRG's lower-than-average length of stay. If, on the other hand, these patients are admitted all over the house in various units, I might question whether or not the nursing staff was familiar enough with these patients to provide effective and efficient nursing care.

2. Staffing on this unit is permanent, consistent, and adequate to provide a safe nurse-to-patient ratio. No agency personnel are used, and overtime is rarely needed. Therefore, I can assume that the high cost is not due to premium dollars. Turnover on this unit is also fairly low, so the cost cannot be related to orientation, education, or downtime. Staffing is also equitable; that is, each day I have approximately the same number and same mix of staff, so that care is equitable on each day.

3. Nursing treatment of these patients is similar to that rendered elsewhere. We do not use any experimental equipment or supplies that are not already included in the DRG rate, so the high cost is not due to treatment methods.

4. Nursing staff provide comprehensive primary nursing care, with the primary nurse providing total nursing care and passive physical therapy. Is the passive physical therapy truly nursing care, or is it within the realm of the physical therapy department? If nursing is conducting physical therapy, is it also maintaining the traction equipment? Is nursing transporting patients to the

physical therapy department for active physical therapy? If nursing is providing some *nonnursing activity,* is it providing other nonnursing services?

Now I have a focus for my study. I can conduct a simple time-and-motion study to determine what nurses actually do for patients in DRG 243.

If I eliminate these nonnursing activities, will the cost of care decrease to within the state norm? Let us look at DRG 122. Here we see, for example, that circulatory disorders with AMI (acute myocardial infarction) in this particular nursing institution has a lower-than-average length of stay and a lower-than-average cost per case. Yet, if we look at the percentage of this DRG that is nursing cost, we find that it is extremely expensive in terms of nursing care, rating 78.63 percent. However, since it is coming in within the standard average nursing cost per case, we know that this is a very efficient DRG within nursing and within this institution. Can we assume, then, that in DRG 122 nursing is, in fact, providing direct nursing care and is not providing nonnursing activities?

Thus, this report has provided me with data for length-of-stay patterns, staffing methodologies, nonnursing indices, and specialization resources—all on one sheet of paper and all relative to other institutions. The inherent potential of this report for nursing management is immeasurable for creative directors of nursing or for those who are not afraid to truly investigate what is happening within their department.

Figure 2 bears out the assumption that I made for DRG 243. Here we clearly see that, although the nursing cost is over the standard, the cost for the diagnostic ancillary departments is well under the state norm. Therefore, is nursing cross-subsidizing other hospital departments? It appears so.

Figure 2. DRG 243.

DRG	Average Length of Stay	Average Nursing Cost Per Case	Average Diagnostic Ancillary Cost Per Case
243 Back Disorders Medical	8.50 (H) 8.75 (S)	368.47 (H) 312.98 (S)	185.60 (H) 225.50 (S)

Nursing = $55.49 disincentive   *Diagnostic Ancillary = $39.90 incentive*

Cross-subsidization ?

When we completed the case-mix nursing-performance study, we found that there was a direct correlation between nursing and ancillary services. For those hospitals in which nursing is well over budget, ancillary services were well under budget. As the gap closed and nursing services came closer to the actual budget figure, so too did the figure for ancillary services. Nurses have known this correlation to be true for years, but now we have statistical data to prove it.

So, you say, all this means is that administrations will take money from nursing and give it to ancillary services to balance everything out. Certainly, that's one very expeditious way to balance the books. But is it both efficient and effective? Directors of nursing service will have to study this closely. For example, if nurses stop doing nonnursing activities, would we need as much nursing staff? Could we use the staff for other nursing activities, such as patient education, that might lower the length of stay, thereby creating more free beds to increase volume? Would this result in more revenue? If you can't totally eliminate nonnursing tasks, could you consider within your institution the option of billing the ancillary service for those things that we do for that service? For instance, if you make, strip, and set beds back up for the admission and discharge of patients, can you bill that amount of time that it takes a nurse to provide that service to the housekeeping department? This can be done by a simple bookkeeping maneuver at year's end.

Nursing directors must constantly question the efficacy of taking the easy way out—cutting or curtailing services—rather than doing the harder job of becoming more efficient by creative management methods. And, perhaps for the first time in nursing's history, we must evaluate the productivity of the nurse with all of the humanistic problems inherent in nursing.

We must also carefully consider areas such as supplies. Do you, as the director of nursing on the new products committee, decide if your hospital uses IVAC or IMED pumps based on time-saving issues for nurses rather than just the dollar figure of the items?

What about such areas as turnover rate? Research has shown us how expensive this is, so what do we do internally to retain staff and thereby decrease the cost of orientation and downtime?

Many administrators do not see the correlation between the cost of nursing care and both personnel policies and the internal socialization process of the hospital. However, we have to face this reality. When an employee is unhappy, discouraged, and/or unsupported, she (or he) will do only what is absolutely necessary to survive in the system. She will not produce, create, innovate, or consider the broader needs of the facility, such as solvency. Paying the additional dollars for a clinical career ladder, for example, may be more cost-effective than paying for continual orientation, overtime, and the use of outside agency staff.

An article in *Hospital Topics* speaks directly to this issue. The authors state:

> The structure of reimbursement acts as a negative incentive for emphasis on efficiency and cost reduction. The hospital administrator has to balance the obvious need for efficiency against the threat of loss of income implied by these actions.

This system places him or her in a strong approach-avoidance conflict in relation to cost reduction. The more he approaches cost reduction, the greater becomes the need to avoid efficiences for fear of reduced third-party payment.[9]

The authors go on to say that

> . . . the hospital administrator ought not to try to manage . . . solely with rational management techniques. . . . The use of intuition may be more important than analytic methods. The administrator's sensitivity to multiple forces, goals, and values may be more valuable than methods of optimizing, allocating, and minimizing.
>
> He . . . needs to break out of habits of thought in which order, stability, and consistency are paramount and needs to be able to tolerate the resulting ambiguity and appreciate the contribution of opposing or contradictory forces. This calls for substantial mental and emotional equanimity, confidence in one's instincts, and flexibility in actions.[10]

Becoming efficient in the utilization of these management reports represents a subtle swing in the organizational structure of most hospitals, for it eliminates the old hierarchy in which the director of nursing service was either in constant confrontation with the fiscal officer (What does he know about nursing care? He should have to work on the unit, then he'll understand) or the paternalism of the fiscal officer, who shared nothing except what he felt the director of nursing needed to know in order to function, which was usually very little (Here's your budget, you're alloted 1 million dollars. I'll send you monthly reports to let you know how much you are spending). Perhaps we need to consider a joint practice committee composed of directors of nursing service sitting together with the fiscal officers of institutions to establish joint practice protocol.

Managing the System

The DRG system demands an interdependence between these two administrators. The management reports can provide parity, especially when you consider that nursing constitutes the greatest percentage of the overall budget.

However, directors of nursing service must learn to speak "fiscalese" so that they can communicate to the lay fiscal director in terms that he understands and can relate to. Or, better yet, consider hiring a vice-president of nursing or assistant director, depending upon your particular structure, who is a fiscal officer for your department alone and who can directly relate in "fiscalese" to the hospital's fiscal director. If you discover, through trends, that you might go over budget if everything remains constant, don't go to your fiscal director and explain where nursing costs have arisen because of the new scope of practice that you've implemented. Since he really didn't know the old practice, explaining a new one is irrevelant. Instead, ask him such questions as: If you lower the length of stay of certain DRGs, can you increase volume significantly to make up the budget deficit? Which DRGs would you have to concentrate

---

[9]E. A. Simendinger, and J. D. Aram, "The Management Job of the Hospital Administrator: Incentive, Dilemma, Contradiction, and Negative," *Hospital Topics,* November-December 1982, p. 5.

[10]*Ibid.,* p. 6.

on increasing? How you decrease the length of stay, such as through a new scope in practice, is up to you and of little interest to him.

What the whole thing comes down to is that nurses must stop being slaves. Don't allow the system to manage you. Learn how to manage the system. To manage the system, you must know and understand it; once it's known, directors of nursing service must demand a voice in decision making. They must be in control of, and therefore accountable for, their budgets, and they must not allow others to determine how much knowledge they need to manage the system.

We also must guard against camouflaging tactics; for example, how often have we heard the following remarks: "I can't give you any additional staff lines because DRG won't allow it," or "If RIMs are implemented, we'll have to cut staff," or "What difference does it make if you transport patients or I hire a transporter; the bottom line is still the same," or "The statistical basis of RIMs is questionable; therefore, it isn't a good indicator of nursing costs," or "RIMs are based on what is, not what should be; therefore, it isn't sensitive to changing trends and certainly disregards quality issues," and so on. I view all of these as scare tactics used to mask the true underlying importance of the system for nursing. What everyone is still afraid of is a mystery to me, and I can only surmise that it is a further and continued attempt to maintain control over nursing. Heaven forbid, the decisions made by a knowledgeable, creative, female director of nursing should turn out to either make or break an institution. Can these crucial decisions really be left in the hands of nurses?

Of equal puzzlement is the fact that progressive administrators don't seem to hold these fears at all. Many have very effectively used their directors of nursing service as partners. For example, one director of nursing service in New Jersey was newly promoted to vice-president, and she has the responsibility of directing both the nursing department and all other ancillary departments as well, thereby both creating a major departure from the traditional hierarchical structure and acknowledging the relationship between these various services.

It is time to work with the DRG system and to recognize that opposition to its principle is self-serving and for the weak-of-heart.

If this sounds like revolution, then I plead guilty for, as Ron Karenga stated, "Revolution is merely creation of an alternative."[11] What is wrong with an alternative to a health care delivery system that consumers are increasingly unable to purchase because of its increasingly high price? What is wrong with an alternative to a system that purpetuates exploitation of labor to such an extent that the labor force flees in droves? What is wrong with an alternative to a system that fosters constraints on creativity, professional growth, and self-actualization? What is wrong with change? What is wrong with challenge?

The challenge is upon us: do we survive the DRG system by making it our slave, or do we fear the risk so much that we retreat and retain our own chains?

---

[11]Brussell. op. cit.. p. 496.

NURSING AND DRGs: PROACTIVE RESPONSES TO PROSPECTIVE REIMBURSEMENT

Jane Meier Hamilton

General systems theory is a study of wholes. It provides us with an organized way to talk about structure and process—what comprises a whole and how it works. A system is any set of interrelated components that interact with each other within a boundary that filters inputs and outputs. Feedback is a mechanism that systems use to correct discrepancies between actual and intended output; it allows systems to be self-directing. In systems, the whole is greater than the sum of its parts; change in one component leads to change in all other components. Finally, all characteristics that apply to systems also apply to their component parts, or subsystems.

Health care in America can be viewed as a system. Subsystems of that whole are innumerable, but those relevant to this article are the nursing profession, the Medicare payment system, health care in the state of New Jersey, and acute-care hospitals.

Let us think of the hospital as a system and the nursing service as one of its many subsystems. The hospital seeks to fulfill its mission of service delivery through the interaction of three kinds of resources (or inputs to the system): human resources (such as staff); technological resources (such as methods and equipment); and financial resources (for example, the operating budget). Each subsystem within the hospital is allocated portions of these resources.[1] Alterations in the amount and type of resources/inputs will lead to changes within the system and each of its subsystems as well.

The amount and type of financial resources available to the American health

---

[1]Ann Butler Maher and Barbara Dolan, "Determining Cost of Nursing Services," *Nursing Management,* 13:9:17, September 1982.

care system have undergone massive changes during the past three decades.
As Spitzer indicates,

> The late 1950s and '60s was a period of building and expansion in the health
> care industry, particularly in acute-care hospitals. National health care policy
> guaranteed access and financial support through the federal government's enact-
> ment of the Hill-Burton Act.... Later in the 1960s, Title XVIII of the Social Securi-
> ty Act was passed, establishing Medicare funding of health care for those over
> 65 years of age. In 1968, the passage of Medicaid (Title XIX) as the state counter-
> part to provide for the indigent led to increased federal support for delivering
> health care for those who could not pay. These changes produced increased de-
> mand and utilization at a time when costs were also rising.
>
> Increases in costs were caused by a variety of factors: inflation, continuing in-
> crease in geriatric and chronically ill populations, increased utilization, inten-
> sification of health services, and increased insurance coverage, to name a few....
> As the government's share of expenses in health care continued to increase, na-
> tional health policy shifted from "guaranteed access" to cost containment in the
> 1970s (and 1980s).[2]

The federal wage and price controls in effect between 1971 and 1974 were
designed to cut inflation throughout the nation. A subgoal was to stabilize the
growth in health care costs, which exceeded the inflation rate of the American
economy. President Carter's proposal, the Hospital Cost Containment Act of
1977 (which never passed), would have been another control measure. It would
have limited the average reimbursement received by hospitals from third-party
payers as well as from self-payers. The 1970s also found the federal government supporting the development of health maintenance organizations as an
approach to preventing serious illness and possibly limiting use of costly hospital
services. Nevertheless, despite all of these attempts at cost control, health care
prices continued to soar.

In the late 1970s, a new approach to health care funding was being developed
at the Yale-New Haven Hospital and, subsequently, at the New Jersey Department of Health. The new approach to cost control, called *prospective payment*,
pays on a cost-per-discharge basis and provides incentives for hospitals to *limit*
costs and to operate efficiently. In 1980, New Jersey began reimbursing 26
hospitals using a form of prospective payment known as the DRG (diagnosis
related group) system.

A dollar figure for each DRG, based on retrospective cost data for a hospital
and region, is derived by averaging the cost of the care given to patients who
have had a specific diagnosis, adjusted to account for inflation. The income
that the hospital will receive for each DRG is determined by multiplying the
average cost times the number of patients that the hospital had discharged who
had been assigned to that DRG.[3]

By 1983, all New Jersey hospitals were being reimbursed according to the
DRG system. During March of that year, the U.S. Congress passed amend-

---

[2]Roxanne B. Spitzer, "Legislation and New Regulations," *Nursing Management*, February 1983.

[3]Leah Curtin, "Determining the Cost of Nursing Services per DRG," *Nursing Management*, 14:4:16, April 1983.

ments to the Social Security Act. Title VI provides for the use of DRG payments for Medicare inpatient hospital services, effective October 1. Though similar in some ways, there are a few differences between the New Jersey and the federal prospective payment systems. In the words of the Commissioner of the New Jersey Department of Health, J. Richard Goldstein,

> ... the New Jersey system is an all-payer system, while the national system will apply only to Medicare. Secondly, there are many items which the New Jersey system provides for which are not provided for in the federal system. For instance, the New Jersey system includes financial elements for uncompensated care, working capital, capital facilities replacement, reimbursement for pediatric conditions or those related to childbirth, and other things.[4]

In New Jersey, all acute-care general hospitals are reimbursed on the basis of DRGs. Under the federal system, most acute-care, short-term, nonfederal hospitals that serve Medicare beneficiaries will be affected. Psychiatric, long-term, children's, and rehabilitation hospitals will be reimbursed under the old system, subject to TEFRA (Tax Equity and Fiscal Responsibility Act) targets. In addition, distinct psychiatric and rehabilitation units of acute-care general hospitals will also be exempt under the federal prospective payment system.

The health care system has had to face some major financial changes in the past 30 years—funding for rapid expansion, soaring health care costs, nationwide inflation, and numerous failed attempts at cost control. These financial changes have been the result of alterations in other components of the health care system (for example, the explosion of medical knowledge and technology, specialization of personnel, and wage demands). Similarly, financial changes have caused alterations in other components of the health care system (such as the growth of HMOs, the development of multihospital systems, and the focus on improving management of health care institutions). As in any system, change in one component will lead to change in all others.

The new prospective payment system is the latest financial change, and its impact will be felt throughout all subunits of the health care system, nursing included. Within hospitals, nursing service is the largest department, and it generally consumes the largest portion of a hospital's budget. Consequently, nursing is particularly vulnerable to cost-containment policies. As case-mix reimbursement is implemented, those who manage nursing service departments will be called upon to operate more efficiently while providing quality patient care. They will have to improve their planning, organizing, staffing, direction, and controlling functions in order to meet this challenge. The following are some specific ways in which nursing will need to respond.

PLANNING

Perhaps the most significant element of the planning function under prospective reimbursement relates to budgeting. Financial resources will become

---

[4]J. Richard Goldstein, "Lessons from the New Jersey Experience: From the Top Down," *Health Care Strategic Management,* October 1983, p. 18.

increasingly scarce and more difficult to obtain. Carolyne K. Davis, administrator of the Health Care Financing Administration (HCFA), states that it will be imperative that nurse administrators and managers develop the skills to forecast departmental needs as well as the knowledge and skills to develop a budget based on forecasted needs. In addition, nurse managers will need solid negotiation skills to ensure the procurement of necessary resources.[5] Elizabeth Buff, vice-president of nursing at the Medical Center at Princeton, says that nurse administrators should learn to talk the financial officer's jargon. It is essential to present nursing needs in the appropriate terminology; take a basic accounting course.[6]

In addition to developing skills for planning nursing service's budget, the vice-president of nursing should be concerned about planning on a hospital-wide basis. She (or he) should be a member of the hospital budget committee as well as any cost-containment committee or any committee that plans the implementation of prospective payment.[7] As the largest component of the hospital system and the major provider of the hospital's health care services, nursing will be affected by, and in some cases will be called upon to implement, administrative plans. The nursing department's understanding of patient needs and the department's own resource needs argue forcefully for nursing to assume a significant role in planning for the distribution of hospital resources.

In addition to planning for the use of resources, nursing must focus renewed attention on the discharge planning process. Because the prospective payment system rewards efficiency, efforts will be made to control the length of stay and to discharge patients as quickly as possible. Effective discharge planning will be an important tool in maintaining quality care in the face of pressures to discharge. A director of nursing at a New Jersey HMO says that fears of endangering patients' safety with inappropriately early discharges have not been realized in New Jersey under DRGs; patients have not been harmed by attempts to control length of stay. Discharge planning is one way in which nurses can transfer the positive results of the New Jersey experience to the national level.

ORGANIZING

Following the first phase of implementing the case-mix reimbursement system in New Jersey, that state's Health Research and Educational Trust (HRET) commissioned DRG evaluation studies. One study examined how the DRG system affects the organization and management of hospitals. Findings show that changes are felt mostly at the departmental and vice-presidential levels.

---

[5]Carolyne K. Davis, "The Federal Role in Changing Health Care Financing," *Nursing Economics,* September/October, 1983, p. 104.

[6]Elizabeth Buff, "The Impact of DRG on Hospital Operations." Speech given at Medicus Conference, Chicago, October 1983.

[7]*Ibid.*

One hypothesis of the HRET study states that the decision-making authority of department heads in DRG hospitals will be larger and that DRG hospitals will be more decentralized as a result. Several aspects of this hypothesis were borne out. Department heads do have a higher level of decision-making authority in DRG hospitals than in non-DRG hospitals. Reciprocal work flow patterns, known to be associated with higher decision-making authority, are found in DRG hospitals, and reciprocal work flow generates some significant departmental characteristics. Members of these departments are more dependent on each other, as well as on the department head, to accomplish necessary tasks. Department heads exert greater influence on departmental operating rules and procedures. The frequency of written and verbal communication is also greater. The reliance on performance standards and evaluations is somewhat higher, though not to a significant degree. Nursing departments, in particular, have operating rules and policies that are more specific and more strictly enforced in DRG hospitals than in their non-DRG counterparts. Decentralization is greater in DRG hospitals, and it is not associated with more conflicts or coordination problems.[8]

Developing a decentralized organizational structure will help the nursing department respond to the challenges of the prospective reimbursement system in several ways.

First, decentralization will diminish the demands on time of the vice-president of nursing, thereby freeing her (or him) to focus on hospital-wide policy issues.

Second, this form of organization will help middle and first-line nurse managers to function truly as managers. It will call on them to monitor departmental and specific unit productivity, quality care, and resource consumption.

Finally, decentralization will push decision-making authority down the organization and involve staff nurse in making decisions about their own jobs and about patient care. This involvement often yields higher levels of productivity, improved quality of output, greater organizational commitment, and better morale.

The sum total of these changes will be more efficient and more effective output from the nursing department, an imperative under the fiscal constraints of DRGs.

STAFFING

One of the most critical problems that a hospital (or nursing) administrator faces is staffing the nursing service. Nursing not only is the most costly single component of hospital operations, but is also has a direct bearing on the quality of care.[9] Total nursing costs—essentially, the salaries and fringe benefits paid

---

[8]Hans Boerma, *"DRG Evaluation Volume IV-B: The Organizational Impact of DRGs"* (Princeton, N.J.: Health Research and Educational Trust of New Jersey at the Center for Health Affairs, 1983) pp. vii-ix, 50-54.

[9]Richard Jelinek and Frank Pierce, "A Nursing System Approach: Productivity and Quality of Care," *Public Productivity Review,* September 1983, p. 223.

to registered nurses, licensed practical nurses, and nurse aides—comprise roughly 30 percent of the typical hospital's budget for direct patient care. Therefore, proper allocation of nursing costs is essential if the hospital's costs are to be measured accurately and managed effectively.[10]

At this time, nursing costs, as a general expense category, are used in the overall development of room rates. Until this time, specific costs of nursing services per patient have never been clearly identified or used to justify nursing's budget or staffing requests. There is a growing need to document the cost of specific health care services, and nursing is no exception. "The new federal regulations do not directly affect reimbursement for nursing services (they are included in the average or target costs), but there is considerable evidence that hospital nursing departments will be required to justify costs for nursing services according to patients' acuity which, in turn, must correlate with the patient's DRG."[11] New Jersey has researched and developed just such a patient classification and cost-justification model, and plans to pilot its use in 1984, with statewide implementation planned for 1985.[12]

The methodology being piloted in New Jersey in 1984 will replace the per diem method of costing out nursing care. It is based on six years of extensive research in three distinct, but related, pilot studies. The fourth study, entitled "The Case-Mix Nursing Performance Study," produced the RIMs methodology. RIMs stands for *relative intensity measures*; they are cost-allocation statistics that specifically relate a patient's consumption of nursing resources to the patient's medical condition. Nursing resources are defined in terms of minutes of nursing care that a patient receives; relative intensity increases as more nursing resources are consumed. As relative intensity increases, so does the cost of nursing care. RIMs were derived mathematically from the analysis of nursing care provided to 2,660 patients on 63,400 shifts between November 1979 and January 1981. The RIMs data were collected in eight New Jersey hospitals, and the relative intensity measures were then developed by researchers for the New Jersey Department of Health.[13]

No other patient classification system has been so extensively studied and, due to the far-reaching implications of this study, none has been so controversial. There are definite limitations to the study in its present form, and more work is required to refine the system. Despite detractions, however, this form provides a more accurate measure of the use of nursing resources than does the per diem method currently in use.

Without a viable patient classification tool, control of staffing and budgeting

---

[10]Paul Grimaldi and Julie Micheleti, "RIMs and the Cost of Nursing Care," *Nursing Management*, 12:12:12, December 1982.

[11]Curtin, *loc. cit.*

[12]J. Richard Goldstein, *Summary of Public Comments and Department Responses Re: N.J.A.C.* 8:31-B.19 Implementation of RIM Methodology (Trenton, N.J.: State of New Jersey Department of Health, July 19, 1982), p.1

[13]*White Paper on the Relative Intensity Measures (RIMs) Methodology Developed by the New Jersey State Department of Health to Incorporate Measures of Nursing Intensity into the Dignosis-Related Group (DRG) Prospective Payment Mechanism* (New York: Deloitte, Haskins and Sells, January 1983), pp.5-7.

could easily be removed from nurses' hands. The impact of this on nursing service and patient care should be considered. Without a patient classification tool, budget and/or staffing cuts will be based on assumptions or, at best, imprecise data. This is not a very sound decision-making strategy. Someone with more power, but not necesarry more accurate data, could make decisions about nursing practice. A valid classification tool, on the other hand, will allow budget and/or staffing decisions to be made on the basis of accurate data by nurses, who know nursing. The latter approach will help to ensure nursing's accountability, implementation of the best possible staffing patterns, and the most effective delivery of nursing care.

DIRECTING

In the area of directing or leading, nursing's response to prospective payment should have a dual focus. First, all nurses should be educated about the prospective payment system and its impact on nursing. Educational sessions should provide technical information about changes in the law; they should also address the behavior and attitude changes that prospective payment will require of nurses.

The traditional nursing role is characterized by a commitment to giving quality care without much concern for the cost of that care. This traditional nursing role is in direct conflict with the current emphasis on the financial aspects of health care. Faced with a conflict between the old "fiscal ignorance" and the new "fiscal responsibility," some nurses will be angry and may resist change.

If nursing service departments are to operate in a cost-effective manner while still providing quality care, this resistance must be overcome. Staff nurses must support and implement nursing management's fiscal policies. To obtain this support, nursing administration must provide a forum for discussing those nursing role changes brought about by the advent of prospective payment. Educational programs must also give nurses the knowledge and the skills required to provide quality care efficiently.

The second element of the directing efforts should focus on nurse managers. As described earlier, decentralization is greater in hospitals receiving prospective reimbursement for health care services. As a result of this, steps should be taken to develop the leadership and managerial skills of first-line nurse managers. The people filling these positions are crucial to the successful operation of nursing service, and because nursing is such a major component of the hospital system, they are crucial to the success of the hospital as a whole. It is through head nurses or nursing unit managers that administration's policies and information are articulated to the staff. Likewise, it is through these first-line managers that the ideas, experiences, and opinions of the staff are communicated to administration. Difficulties in fulfilling managerial functions at this level of the organization will have a negative impact on productivity, morale, implementation of change, quality of care, and the cost of nursing operations.

Management education program should be offered to nurse managers on an ongoing basis; in addition, an orientation to the management role and job functions should be offered to each new nurse manager. Educational programs should have a very practical focus, providing skills that nurse managers can use in their day-to-day operations.

Nurse managers need to develop skills in all management functions. They should learn the skills of staffing and scheduling, with special attention paid to linking these with patient acuity. They should learn how to prepare a budget and how to control costs at the unit level. They should learn how to assess the productivity of their unit and how to motivate their staff to function in a highly productive manner. They should learn how to develop and achieve unit, as well as individual, objectives. Finally, they should learn how to delegate, solve problems, implement change, and resolve conflicts. First-line nurse managers are key figures in any nursing organzation. The importance of their role will only increase as hospitals and their nursing service departments face the challenge of the prospective payment system.

CONTROLLING

Due to the fact that case-mix reimbursement is an attempt to control health care costs, most of the responses to this payment mechanism serve a controlling function. Many of the responses previously described, particularly the budget and the patient classification system, are controls. In addition to these, there are three additional recommendations for controlling nursing service under DRGs.

First, nursing should actively pursue acquisition of a computer information system, if one is not already in place, that integrates management and patient care information. With prospective payment comes a growing demand for accurate and complete documentation of services and costs. As health care becomes increasingly complex, caregivers and managers will become more dependent on one another for information to control patient care and management operations. Requests for data to justify, document, analyze, and forecast are growing at an astronomical rate, and it appears that this trend will continue. On-line interactive computer systems are, at present, the most efficient method of addressing this need. When these routine data-processing operations are computerized, professionals are freed for more creative effort, and nursing service can operate more productively.

Nurses use, gather, and generate large volumes of data that must be shared with others. These data are both clinical and managerial in nature. When planning for adoption of a computer information system in nursing, this should be taken into account. Choice of a system that can integrate both clinical and managerial data would be most forward thinking; such a system would respond best to the information and control needs of nursing. Adoption of any computer information system will require careful planning, and nurses should have input into the choice or design of software. Staff will require educational support both before and during adoption of computer services.

Second, nursing service should regularly gather departmental statistics and develop meaningful reports. In order to function effectively, nurse managers and administrators must possess a wide variety of information about the personnel and operations of the nursing department. This information must be current, clearly organized, and readily available to nursing and hospital leaders. Without accessible, accurate data, nursing management breaks down. Planning, organizing, leading, staffing, and controlling functions are all undermined. A few examples of data that should be collected on a regular basis are nurse-to-patient ratios, occupancy of each unit, hours of nursing care expended on each unit, budget data, patient acuity linked to staffing data turnover rates, salary data, and productivity data for all units.

Finally, nursing service should take definitive steps to control nursing staff involvement in nonnursing functions. One vice-president of nursing in New Jersey says that under DRGs nursing service loses money when providing services other than direct patient care. Transport of patients and materials, housekeeping chores, and some clerical functions are considered nonnursing functions. Under DRGs, nursing receives minimal reimbursement for these services; DRGs provide an incentive for nurses to perform nursing duties. Nonnursing functions should be delegated or assigned to appropriate staff—either paid or voluntary personnel.

Thus, the health care industry today is a system in transition. New prospective payment guidelines are designed to control costs in the health care system in general and in hospitals specifically. The largest labor and financial component of any hospital is its nursing service. Therefore, the efficiency of nursing operations will be a key determinant of the success or failure of any hospital's cost-containment efforts. If quality of care is not to suffer under cost containment, nursing service must be well managed.

In order to survive and thrive under the new prospective payment system, nursing must not assume a passive stance and wait for others to dictate nursing's response. Nursing itself must take proactive steps to respond to the pressures of prospective reimbursement. By implementing the planning, organizing, staffing, directing, controlling measures outlined in this article, nursing will prepare itself to meet the challenges of the new system.

DRGs:
REGULATORY ADJUSTMENTS

James M. Gaynor, Jr., Dean A. Kant,
and Elizabeth M. Mills

The Social Security Admendments of 1983, signed into law on April 20, 1983, established a national prospective payment system (PPS) for Medicare inpatient hospital care. Final regulations implementing PPS have now been issued. Many hospitals came under implementing PPS have now been issued. Many hospitals came under PPS on October 1, 1983, and all hospitals that are subject to PPS will come unde it by October 1, 1984.

The purpose of prospective payment are to simplify the method of determining the payment amount to a hospital for services rendered to Medicare beneficiaries and to control Medicare costs by setting, in advance, the amount that will be paid for care. Hospitals (theoretically) will have an incentive to control their costs because, if their costs are lower than the prospective payment, they may keep the difference. Conversely, if their costs are higher, hospitals will lose money. Under the former system of reasonable-cost reimbursement, hospitals had no incentive to control costs or volume of services because (within broad limits) all costs incurred were reimbursed.

While PPS is simple in theory, its implementation is complicated, and the need to phase in PPS in a way that will avoid disruption of hospital care introduces additional complexities. This paper summarizes PPS, how payment amounts are calculated, and the additional scrutiny to which hospitals will be subjected with PPS.

BOUNDARIES OF PROSPECTIVE PAYMENT

For hospitals subject to PPS, payment for each Medicare discharge in cost-reporting periods beginning on or after October 1, 1983, will be computed under PPS. The full PPS amount is paid for each stay during which there is at least one covered Medicare day of care. Payment is calculated by multiplying a standard rate per discharge by the DRG weight assigned to that discharge. This

109

payment covers inpatient operating costs for that discharge. The PPS amount includes the costs of nonphysician services that previously could be billed by a nonhospital supplier under Part B of the Medicare program (for example, laboratory services supplied by a clinical laboratory, for which the patient was billed directly by the laboratory).

Specifically, effective for services provided on or after October 1, 1983, PPS prohibits the "unbundling" of hospital services; that is, the costs of all non-physician services provided to hospital patients will be reimbursed only to the hospital. Nonphysician services are defined in the regulations as all hospital services except physicians' services. Physicians services are services that: are personally furnished to an individual patient by a physician; contribute directly to the diagnosis or treatment of an individual patient; ordinarily require performance by a physician; and, if the physician is an anethesiologist, radiologist, or pathologist, meet additional requirements enumerated in the regulations.

The unbundling prohibition means that, where services are funished under arrangements to hospital inpatients, the supplying organization must now accept its payment from the hospital. The term "under arrangements" refers to a manner of arranging to have (other than physicians') services furnished by a supplier or provider outside the hospital. The amount charged by the supplying organization and paid by the hospital is a cost to the hospital. If the hospital is not paid under PPS, these costs are to be included in its cost report. If the hospital is on a prospective-rate basis, the prospective payment is deemed to include payment for services furnished under specific arrangements.

In accordance with the theoretical underpinnings of PPS, a hospital is prohibited from charging a beneficiary for services paid under PPS, even if the hospital's costs for the services exceed the amount paid. However, under circumstances defined in the regulations, a hospital may charge a beneficiary for applicable deductible and coinsurance amounts; custodial care; medically unnecessary items and services requested by the patient; and customary charge differentials for private rooms or other luxury items more expensive than those medically required.

Not included in the prospective payment amount, but paid for separately, are outpatient services, direct and indirect medical education costs, outlier costs, and capital-related costs. At least through 1986, capital-related costs will be reimbursed on a reasonable-cost basis. Therefore, successful classification of costs as capital-related will result in higher payments to hospitals. Capital-related costs generally include depreciation expenses, property taxes, lease and rental payments, interest expense for acquiring assets, and return on equity capital for proprietary providers. The standards used by a hospital for classifying costs as capital items or as operating expenses under PPS must be consistent with the standards that the hospital used before PPS.

Outlier payments are designed to protect from financial hardship hospitals treating extraordinarily costly cases. Outliers are cases within a particular DRG that have unusually long lengths of stay ("day outliers") or unusually high costs ("cost outliers"). However, outlier payments will not necessarily compensate hospitals for the full cost of care and treatment, for they will approximate only the marginal cost of care beyond the specified outlier threshold criteria (days or dollar amounts).

A day outlier is a case in which the length of stay (LOS) exceeds the LOS for the applicable DRG by the lesser of (a) a fixed number of days, as specified by HCFA, or (b) a fixed number of standard deviations from the mean LOS for the applicable DRG, also as specified by HCFA. In 1984, the threshold criteria are 20 days or 1.94 standard deviations. HCFA will update the threshold criteria in an annual notice.

A cost outlier is a case in which the cost of covered services exceeds the greater of (a) a fixed dollar amount (adjusted for local wages), as specified by HCFA; or (b) a fixed multiple of the prospective payment rate for the applicable DRG. In 1984, the threshold criteria are $12,000 or 1.5. Again, HCFA will update the threshold criteria in an annual notice.

A hospital need not specifically request payment for day outliers, as such payment will be made automatically for medically necessary days along with payment for the discharge. The same is not true for cost outliers.

CALCULATION OF PROSPECTIVE PAYMENT AMOUNTS

After a three-year transition period, prospective payment will be based on an annually determined standard payment amount per discharge ("federal national rate"). There will be one standard amount for urban hospitals and a separate standard amount for rural hospitals. The rate that each hospital actually receives will be adjusted for local wage variations. The standard amount adjusted for local wage variations is multiplied by the DRG weighting factors to determine the payment in a specific case. Except for the wage and urban-rural differences, payment for discharges falling into the same DRG will be the same for every hospital in the United States.

To minimize substantial disruptions in reimbursement levels, PPS will be phased in over a three-year period, beginning with each hospital's first cost-reporting period starting after September 1983. During the transition period, payment will be based in part on federal rates and in part on hospital-specific rates, which are based on individual hospitals' cost experiences. In turn, federal rates will be based partly on national rates and partly on regional rates, with rates for each of nine census regions.

Payments will be made as follows during this three-year period: In the first year, 25 percent of the payment will be based on regional rates and 75 percent on each hospital's hospital-specific rate; in the second year, 50 percent of the payment will be based on a combination of national and regional rates (25 percent national and 75 percent regional) and 50 percent of the payment will be based on the hospital-specific rate; and in the third year, 75 percent of the payment will be based on a combination of national and regional rates (50 percent national and 50 percent regional) and 25 percent of the payment will be based on the hospital-specific rate. In the fourth year (beginning on or after October

1, 1986), the program will be fully phased in, and payment will be based entirely on the above-described national payment rates.

The hospital-specific rate, which plays a descreasing role in payment throughout the transition period, is based on a hospital's costs per Medicare discharge in the base year (the cost-reporting period ending before September 30, 1983). Base year costs are adjusted so that the costs included correspond to the costs that are to be covered under the prospective payment amount (capital and medical education costs are removed) and are adjusted by a case-mix index developed for each hospital. This standardized cost per Medicare discharge for the hospital is multiplied by an updating factor (which contains inflation factors) to bring costs up to 1984, and a budget neutrality factor.

The inflation factors are based on projected inflation in the goods and services that hospitals purchase (the hospital market basket), plus a small additional allowance. The result is the hospital-specific rate. For subsequent cost-reporting periods during the transition period, the hospital-specific rate will be updated using target-rate inflation factors and recalculated budget-neutrality factors, if applicable.

Because hospital-specific rates are based on costs allowed in the base year, changes in allowed costs will result in changes in the hospital-specific rate. For example, after a successful appeal of cost disallowances related to the base period, the intermediary will have to recalculate the hospital-specific rate, including the cost found to be allowed. The adjusted rate will be effective only for cost-reporting periods beginning after the appeal decision date; retroactive revision of the hospital-specific rate will not be made. On the other hand, if it is later determined that costs in the base year were fraudulently claimed, the hospital-specific rate will be recalculated and all excess prospective payments recovered.

Until 1986, 18 regional standard rates will be calculated each year, one for urban areas and one for rural areas of each of the nine census regions. For fiscal year (FY) 1984, these rates are based on the allowable Medicare operating costs (excluding medical education and capital costs) and discharges contained in all hospital cost reports for reporting periods ending in 1981. Allowable costs are standardized for local wages and case-mix indices, adjusted by actual and projected inflation factors to project the amounts forward to 1984, and adjusted for a budget-neutrality factor. The costs per discharge are then aggregated into the 18 standardized rates per discharge (the federal standard rates).

Both during and after the transition period, the portion of the prospective payment amount based on federal standard rates will be adjusted for local hospital wages. HCFA will compute a wage adjustment factor for each standard metropolitan area and a single factor for all rural areas of each state. These factors are based on Bureau of Labor Statistics (BLS) data on wages paid by hospitals in each area.

The wage adjustment can have a large impact on the amount of prospective payment that hospitals receive. The wage index could reduce the federal portion of prospective payment to a hospital to 80 percent of the published rate or increase it to 137 percent of the rate. The importance of wage adjustment will increase in future years, as more of a hospital's actual payment is based on the federal rate and less on the hospital-specific rate. Congress mandated this adjustment to prevent hardship for hospitals in high wage areas and windfalls for hospitals in low wage areas. There have been complaints that the BLS data are not appropriate for calculating wage indices. For example, the data do not differentiate between full-time and part-time employees, so that hospitals paying the same hourly wage but with different proportions of part-time employees would have different indices. Also, hospitals outside of designated metropolitan areas must use statewide indices, which may not reflect local labor market conditions. Relief for rural hospitals is currently being considered by Congress.

HCFA will calculate the budget neutrality factor by estimating the total Medicare payments for a fiscal year that would have been paid under the old reimbursement system and which will be paid under prospective payment. To the extent that its estimates show more payments under PPS, the payment rates for all hospitals under PPS will be reduced so that estimated expenditures under either approach will be equal. Therefore, not only is a hospital's prospective payment not necessarily related to its actual costs of providing care to Medicare patients, but also, in the aggregate, reimbursement under PPS is not guaranteed to cover total hospital costs incurred for serving Medicare patients nationally.

EXCLUSIONS AND SPECIAL TREATMENT
UNDER PROSPECTIVE PAYMENT

Generally speaking, acute-care hospitals are subject to prospective payment. Children's hospitals, long-term-care hospitals, psychiatric hospitals, rehabilitation hospitals, and alcohol- and drug-treatment hospitals are excluded from PPS. Psychiatric, rehabilitation, and alcohol-and-drug-treatment units of acute-care hospitals that are operated as distinct units are also excluded from prospective payment. (To be a distinct unit, the unit must have beds that are physically separate from those in the rest of the hospital, as well as separately identified admission and discharge records.) Services provided in excluded hospitals and hospital units will be paid for on the current reasonable-cost basis, subject to limits on the rate of cost increases from one year to the next. The regulations set forth detailed criteria that the above-identified hospitals and hospital units must meet in order to be excluded from PPS. A hospital's or hospital unit's status will be determined at the beginning of each cost-reporting period, and this status will generally apply throughout said period.

In addition, the regulations provide that states with cost-control programs may apply to HCFA for a Medicare waiver that, if approved, will result in hospitals in those states being paid under those programs and not under PPS. A state may receive a waiver if its cost-control program applies to all hospitals in the state; treats payors, hospital employees, and patients equitably; and will not result in higher Medicare costs.

Several types of hospitals paid under PPS will receive special treatment. The most significant of these is the sole-community hospital (SCH). An SCH is a hospital that qualifies as the sole source of inpatient hospital services to Medicare beneficiaries in a geographic area. A hospital wishing to qualify as an SCH must be in a rural area and must be either more than 50 miles from another hospital or between 15 and 50 miles from other hospitals, and must meet other criteria indicating isolation. An SCH will receive payment at 75 percent of the hospital-specific rate and 25 percent of the federal rate for all future cost-reporting periods. The hospital-specific payment portion will not be phased out as it will be for other hospitals; thus, payment will continue to be based partly on the hospital's own costs. An SCH can also receive additional payments during the three-year transition period if its total discharges decrease by more than 5 percent due to extraordinary, externally imposed circumstances beyond its control.

TRANSFERS

PPS currently makes a distinction between patients who are "discharged" and patients who are "transferred." A patient is discharged when he is formally released from a hospital, dies, or is transferred to another hospital or unit excluded from the system. A patient is transferred when he is moved from one PPS-paid hospital to another such hospital or to a hospital excluded from prospective payment because it is under a waivered state program or it has not yet entered prospective payment. HCFA's goal in connection with transfers is to make one payment for all inpatient services associated with a particular diagnosis. However, HCFA has adopted an interim policy of making two payments.

In cases involving transfers, as defined above, payment to the final discharging hospital is made at the full prospective-payment rate. The transferring hospital is paid a per diem rate for the days that the patient was hospitalized in the transferring hospital. This amount cannot exceed the prospective-payment amount that would have been paid if the transferring hospital had discharged the patient. To calculate the per diem payment amount, the full prospective-payment amount for that discharge from the transferring hospital is divided by the average LOS for the DRG in which the patient is included and is then multiplied by the number of days of care actually provided. If treatment is provided under different DRGs at different hospitals, each hospital's payment will be calculated based on the DRG under which the patient was treated at that hospital. No outlier payment will be made to the transferring hospital, but the discharging hospital will be eligible for outlier payments based on the length or cost of the stay in that hospital alone.

REVIEWS AND APPEALS

PPS somewhat curtails administrative and judicial review. Calculation of the amount of payment due under PPS obviously involves complicated calculations and the use of discretion by HCFA in choosing calculation methods. If each hospital could challenge each issue, the purpose of PPS would be defeated because rates would be changing constantly and could not be set in advance. Congress believed that the necessity of maintaining a workable system must preclude review of issues such as the level of prospective payment, the establishment of diagnosis-related groups, the methodology for classifying discharges within such groups, and the appropriate weighting of such groups.

Nonetheless, review is not totally foreclosed. Issues still subject to review include: denial of exclusion from prospective payment as a psychiatric, rehabilitation, or alcohol- and drug-treatment hospital or distinct hospital unit; denial of a special payment basis as an SCH; and disputes regarding items reimbursed on a reasonable-cost basis or outside the prospective payment amount (for example, outlier payments and medical education costs). Limited appeal rights are also available to challenge the calculation of the hospital-specific rate.

One important issue that is still unclear is whether relief after a successful appeal of some issues will be retrospective (all additional payment due since the time of the error will be paid) or only prospective (that is, payment will be increased from the date of the appeal decision or in the next cost-reporting period). Since the appeals process may take several years, the difference is significant.

PROFESSIONAL REVIEW ORGANIZATIONS (PRO) AND DRG VALIDATION

Hospitals must contract with a PRO as a condition precedent to receiving prospective payments. The PRO will review the validity of the diagnostic information furnished, the completeness and adequacy of the care provided, the appropriateness of the admissions and discharges, and the appropriateness of the care supplied to outlier patients.

HCFA may impose penalties if it determines on the basis of PRO-supplied information that a hospital has engaged in unacceptable admissions or inappropriate practices so as to circumvent PPS. HCFA may disallow payment for unacceptable admissions, or it may require the hospital to take corrective action to prevent or correct the inappropriate practices.

PPS requires the fiscal intermediary to assign a hospital discharge to a single DRG, based upon information abstracted from the inpatient bill, regardless of the number of conditions treated or services furnished during the patient's stay. The abstracted information includes principal diagnosis (that is, the diagnosis established after study to be chiefly responsible for occasioning the patient's admission to the hospital), secondary diagnosis, age, sex, procedures performed, and discharge destination. To ensure the accuracy of the abstracted information, a medical review agent (usually a PRO) will review samples of discharges every quarter to ensure that the diagnostic and procedural coding used to assign the DRG are substantiated by the medical records. In addition, with regard to each Medicare discharge, the attending physician must sign the following statement:

> I certify that the identification of the principal and secondary diagnoses and the procedures performed is accurate and complete to the best of my knowledge. (Notice: Intentional misrepresentaton, concealment, or falsification of this information may, in the case of a Medicare beneficiary, be punishable by imprisonment, fine or civil penalty.)

Once the intermediary assigns the discharge to a DRG, it determines the proper prospective payment and pays the hospital.

CONCLUSION

Congress' primary goal in enacting PPS was to create incentives for hospitals to operate in a more efficient and effective manner. It is certain that, in the next few years, the system will undergo changes, but only time will tell whether it will be successful in achieving legislative intent.

DRGs: A MEDICAL RECORDS PERSPECTIVE

Sonja P. Bennett

The challenge of Pubic Law 98-21, the Tax Equity and Fiscal Responsibility Act (TEFRA), is now facing the nation. This law provides Medicare payment for hospital inpatient services under a prospective payment system. This challenge has already been faced and met in New Jersey.

New Jersey hospitals have been phased into the DRG (diagnosis related group) system since 1980. At Riverview Medical Center, we have been submitting the UB (uniform bill) using classification and terminology consistent with the ICD 9 CM (international classification of diseases) and the UHDDS (uniform hospital discharge data set) for the past two years.

The uniform bill is based on the DRG provided by the medical record department. Per diem charging is the system with which we are familiar. It was believed, however, that per diem charging did not measure the hospital's case mix (cases grouped by shared characteristics).

I shall relate certain aspects of this system and how it has made a change in New Jersey, and compare it with the federal plan. I will also discuss our experiences in medical records and with the nursing and medical staffs.

In both the New Jersey and the federal systems, there are 23 MDCs (medical diagnostic categories), in which there are 467 DRGs. The theory behind the DRG system is that patients with similar medical/surgical conditions tend to use similar hospital resources. The objective is to pay hospitals for the health care resources that the category consumes. In New Jersey, the base year costs for 1984 are actually the 1982 costs plus an inflation, or economic, factor. The economic factor is based not only on costs in New Jersey, but on costs in the northeastern region of the United States.

Changes have occurred in all departments, but most predominantly in the medical record department. An expanded role and added responsibilities for the medical record staff have evolved. Reliability of data has become a prime concern. Coding, analyzing, and abstracting the medical record must be done accurately. For proper DRG assignment, medical record personnel require complete diagnoses from physicians. For example, if the patient has thrombophlebitis, the physician should state whether or not it is the deep-vein type; if the patient has renal colic due to renal calculus, both diagnoses should be documented.

Articles have been published concerning the "DRG creep"—the concept that medical records departments are maximizing diagnoses to obtain a higher rate for their patients. True, medical records personnel must closely analyze records to ascertain that all diagnoses and procedures are documented and coded. However, the principal diagnosis—which is the diagnosis established, after study, to be chiefly responsible for occasioning the hospitalization—cannot be changed. In New Jersey, as it will be nationally, audits are conducted to validate appropriate coding and proper DRG assignment. As an example, in a 400-500 bed hospital, such as our medical center, the PRO (professional review organization) audits 125 records, and abstracts and bills quarterly to ensure that proper coding, abstracting, and billing are accomplished.

The timeliness of the physician in completing the record and the need for computerizing medical and financial information must be addressed. In order to generate the DRG, some type of computer capability is necessary, which can be accomplished by an inhouse computer system or by an outside firm. Medical record personnel are responsible for controlling the data, and the uniform bill cannot be generated without the DRG assignment.

With the start of the DRG program, cooperation by the physician has become one of the most important links to reimbursement. There are no physician fees included in the DRG rate unless the physician is salaried or is under contract for services. The DRG is derived from physician information in the medical record, which is why timeliness of completion is important. The physician must be taught to document, on admission, the principal diagnosis and all other diagnoses for which the patient is being treated and, at the time of discharge, any complications and all procedures that occurred. Failure to do this can hinder the cash flow and escalate costs in the medical record and financial departments. TEFRA also requires that physicians verify the principal diagnosis; this requires prompt and complete documentation.

Increased use of same-day surgical units has been urged by the New Jersey Department of Health, which has set a policy for hospitals to follow. A specific list of qualifying procedures was distributed. Included on the list were 7 procedures for orthopedic surgery (for example, diagnostic arthroscopy, ganglionectomy); 20 procedures for plastic and general surgery (for instance, revision of scar, incision and drainage); 10 procedures for urology (for example, circumcision on patients less than one year of age; meatotomy); 20 procedures for gynecology (such as D&C; biopsy of the cervix); 13 procedures for otolaryngology (for instance, myringotomy; tonsillectomy and adenoidectomy); 7 procedures for neurology and neurosurgery (such as decompression of the median nerve; muscle biopsy); and 9 procedures for medicine (for example, thoracentesis; transfusions). In some instances, it may become necessary for patients to be admitted following the procedure. If so, the reasons must be documented by the physician.

Educating physicians to the DRG system was accomplished in New Jersey by various methods: seminars, inservice programs at the various physician section meetings, face-to-face meetings with the director of medical records, and establishment of a DRG committee or a physician DRG liaison who could aid in any hospital/physician problems.

DRGs are aimed at changing physician practice habits. Some physicians treat a given illness at a higher cost than do their peers. With the management reports that are derived from the system, the differences can be identified and the reasons for the differences addressed. Hospitals now look more closely at the ways in which specific diseases are being treated. Physician ordering patterns are scrutinized. Comparative data can be generated, and variations in lengths of stay can be studied.

The Medical Society of New Jersey has questioned whether the DRG system is actually cutting costs or whether it may be eroding the quality of hospital care and enhancing the possibility that patients may be discharged too soon. A bill was filed in the New Jersey assembly to create a committee to study the DRG system. It stated that: There is concern that cost rather than quality of patient care has become a major consideration, and that increases in the number of patients who have died or suffered a relapse soon after their hospital discharge may possibly be linked to premature discharges or lower quality care.

The bill further states that a 13-member committee should be established to study the DRG system in order to determine if this method is contributing to a depreciation in the quality of medical care in hospitals and to evaluate whether the present system should be continued.

In 1984, it became mandatory for New Jersey hospitals to include on the uniform bill whether or not the patient had been discharged from the hospital within the past seven days of his or her latest admission. A study was conducted at our medical center on seven-day readmissions for a three-month period in 1984 to verify if patients actually were being prematurely discharged and had thereby expired or suffered a relapse. Review of readmissions did not reveal this phenomenon.

Not only are physicians involved in questioning the system, but the American Hospital Association in exploring specific DRG price blending. National urban and rural pricing does not take into account hospital cost variations, geographic location, severity of illness, and nonpayments. The hospitals also seek a more equitable system of establishing Medicare prices. Unlike TEFRA, New Jersey's DRG system guarantees full payment for indigent care, debt service payer equity and, thus, aids in eliminating hospital disadvantages.

Our medical center was chosen as one of the hospitals to test RIMs (relative intensity measures) in 1984. This system was developed by the New Jersey State Department of Health in 1980. Since the DRG rates do not accurately reimburse for nursing care, a new method of accounting for nursing services was sought. Patient days are used in New Jersey to allocate nursing care received, but this method ignores the intensity of care and does not adequately reflect per-case resource consumption. Inconsistency in allocating nursing costs can have financial consequences for hospitals and can complicate the nursing director's ability to staff units adequately and in a cost-effective manner. It is thought that RIMs can provide a management tool that will aid in staffing. It is more likely that the federal Medicare program will be looking to New Jersey for insight and guidance on the nursing cost issue.

Since DRGs, closer relationships have developed within hospital departments. The main alliance has been between the medical record and the financial departments. The cash flow is dependent upon our information, which must be accurate and timely. A closer relationship has also developed between nursing and medical record personnel. Several New Jersey hospitals have already developed a program whereby medical record personnel are sent to the floors to audit records while the patient is in house. Dialogue between the nursing staff and medical record personnel is important to ensure that reports are current. Nurses can also facilitate contact with the physician, which is needed in obtaining information for the DRG.

Basically, a flow sheet is developed that is appended to the chart. Medical record personnel perform an ongoing review, coding the diagnoses and procedures and adding any diagnoses gleaned from the physician's notes. By discharge, all information needed for DRG assignment should have been documented. Also, at any given time during the patient's stay, the diagnoses and procedures can be fed into the computer to obtain a DRG and length of stay. This information can be valuable to the financial department to determine the case mix and cash flow.

Implementation of the prospective payment system is not easy. There are many differences between the New Jersey system and TEFRA. The federal plan will not allow hospitals to recover the cost of treating uninsured patients. TEFRA divides the United States into nine regions, splits those into urban and rural categories and, in each of 18 subdivisions, average cost-per-case is the same. The plan is to phase out the regional variations within four years. Outliers will not be treated the same way. In New Jersey, outliers are patients who have been transferred, signed out against medical advice, transferred to another acute care institution, died, or are unusual, atypical cases. About 30 percent of the New Jersey patients are classified as outliers; only an estimated 5 percent are classified for the TEFRA plan.

To be effective under heavy regulation, there must be team effort in all hospital departments. It is important to remember that the care of the patient is still the primary focus of the hospital. Whether, after evaluation, DRG is the best solution for containing health care costs, only time will tell.

SHOULD PATIENT CARE REVENUES BE USED TO EDUCATE HEALTH PROFESSIONALS?

Ruth Hanft

INTRODUCTION

The health sector of the economy is undergoing rapid changes. The expansionist era of the sixties and seventies is over. Fears of shortage and underservice and policies to ameliorate shortages have been replaced by concerns about surplus of manpower, excess facilities and service capacity, and overutilization of services. Major efforts are being made to slow growth. In the sixties and seventies, the federal government and the states deliberately supported the expansion of health professions education of all types. In nursing there was a dramatic shift away from diploma education to baccalaureate and associate degree programs. State governments encouraged the development of RN-to-baccalaureate-degree programs. The federal government stimulated the expansion of master's programs and the development of nurse practitioner and nurse administrator programs. In addition, the federal government supported the development of doctoral programs in nursing.

The sixties and seventies saw the rapid expansion of health financing and service programs: Medicare, Medicaid, community health centers. Hospital facilities and technology expanded rapidly.

The era of the eighties and nineties will probably be characterized by retrenchment and conflict related to financing, service delivery, and education. Some early examples of the changes that are occurring are:

- Increased requirements in public and private insurance for cost sharing by beneficiaries and retrenchment in public health-care programs—Medicare, Medicaid, community and public health;

- Major change in reimbursement for hospital care placing pressure on hospitals to control and/or reduce use of services, staffing, and education programs;

- Unbundling of hospital services and emergence of new outpatient modalities of care including more home-based and freestanding services such as diagnostic testing, total parenteral nutrition, dialysis, respiratory therapy;

- Change from perception of shortages to perception of surplus of manpower in many fields, most notably dentistry, medicine, and now nursing;

- Development of competition and price consciousness with increased enrollment in HMOs and growth of preferred provider arrangements;

- Increased competition among health professionals affecting nurse midwives, nurse anesthetists, nurse clinicians;

- Reduction and termination of federal programs to support health professions education and reductions in state support;

- Pressures to reduce the patient care support for education programs.

It is this last issue that I've been asked to address. In order to do so, it is important first to describe the history of patient care support of health professions education and the effects the changing environment will have on this support.

SUPPORT OF HEALTH PROFESSIONS EDUCATION

Health professions education is supported through multiple financing streams and is distinguished from other higher education programs by its cost and use of patient care funds. All past studies indicate that health professions education is more expensive than other graduate and undergraduate fields, primarily because of the clinical requirements and the low faculty-to-student ratios. It is the clinical requirements that have led to support for education through patient care payments. These payments were originally based on a *quid pro quo,* services provided to patients by the students. The degree of patient care support varies widely by each health profession and site of training.

In most other fields of higher education, support is provided by the following financing streams: state support for state colleges and universities; tuition; endowment funds; and grants and contracts for research, which range from negligible in the humanities, through small sums in the social sciences, to substantial support in many of the sciences, particularly biomedical fields.

Only in the health professions have substantial, and until recently growing, amounts of support come from the provision of service to population groups—patient care funds. These patient care funds are provided in several ways. A hospital pays stipends to certain types of students, mainly medical and dental residents. Hospital salaries support faculty, most commonly in medicine, dentistry, clinical pharmacy, and in some hospital-based training programs in nursing and allied health. Hospitals and other agencies contribute costs for classroom space, supplies, staff of the institution who supervise students, etc. Fees are generated by faculty for patient care services, most commonly in medicine and dentistry.

No one has yet accounted for the total costs of education borne by patient care revenues, particularly hospital revenues. Furthermore, when public policy officials speak of teaching hospitals they are describing only the hospitals with approved medical residency programs. Yet we are all aware of numerous hospitals without residencies in medicine, yet which do provide the clinical laboratory for training nurses, social workers, and allied health personnel, and of other agencies like visiting nurse services and public health clinics which also provide support.

Before discussing the rationale for the use of patient care funding and the changes that may be imminent, I'd like to describe briefly the support of nursing education at all levels.

SUPPORT OF NURSING EDUCATION

There are different streams of support and degrees of support for different types of nurse training and for different terminal degrees. Where once a large proportion of nursing education was financed by patient care revenues, when diploma education was predominant, this balance has shifted substantially to support from states and tuition.

Associate Degree: Initially associate degree programs were supported almost exclusively through state and local revenues that underwrite community colleges and tuition. There was considerable criticism that many of these programs were not providing sufficient clinical experience, and hospital administrators claimed that they had to provide further training for many of the graduates. In recent years, particularly during the period of the shortage of nurses, hospitals began to develop close clinical relationships with community colleges and indirectly supported the clinical training by contributing space and staff supervision.

Diploma Nursing: The three-year hospital-based programs have declined rapidly. Those that remain still receive the majority of support from their hospital base, but have increasingly become linked with community colleges and baccalaureate programs.

Baccalaureate Nursing: The non-nursing portion of baccalaureate nursing programs is supported through state appropriations and tuition. The clinical portions receive support similar to other nursing and allied health clinical programs, mainly, space and staff supervision from health care agencies. Faculty is supported from college and university sources of revenue.

Master's Nursing Programs: Support depends on the nature and clinical orientation of the programs. Faculty in nursing administratin and other nonclinical nurse specialties are supported in the same way as most other higher education programs, except that federal funds, now declining, helped support and expand these programs. Some nursing faculty also receive support through research grants but in substantially lesser amounts than medicine, dentistry, or pharmacy.

Doctoral Programs: Most of these programs were started with direct federal funding. Since the majority of the few doctoral programs are designed to produce faculty and researchers, there is little support from third-party payers. Some, but modest, research funding has begun to flow to schools with doctoral programs.

Several factors distinguish nursing education from other health professions education, particularly medicine and dentistry. In a number of baccalaureate and master's programs in nursing, students study part-time for financial reasons and support themselves by actually practicing their profession. Tuition in nursing schools represents a higher proportion of education costs than in medicine or dentistry. In addition, faculty salaries in nursing are lower than those in many academic fields. To maintain skills and augment income, faculty often work as part-time nurses and are paid for service, *not* education, activities by a hospital or other agency.

In a few nursing programs based in academic health centers, where the Rochester model is used, nursing faculty receive part of their salary from the teaching hospital, but again for service not teaching. By and large, full-time nursing faculty do not receive support from patient care funds.

A few nursing schools have attempted to form faculty practice plans similar to those of medicine and dentistry. However, since few nurses are able to bill on a fee-for-service basis, these plans do not generate large amounts of income.

ISSUES IN PATIENT CARE FINANCING OF
HEALTH PROFESSIONS EDUCATION

Most of the questions of financing of health professions education through patient care funding have focused on medicine and on four issues: (1) Whether society should subsidize the training of MDs, the highest earning profession, more generously than other fields; (2) the distributive inequity of this support on patients and regions of the country; (3) the escalating cost of health care and the need to control all factors that contribute to the increase in cost; and (4) distortions in training that have developed due to financing incentives leading to specialty imbalances.

Support of the Highest Earning Profession

Medical education is heavily subsidized. Tuition, except in a few institutions, represent a lower portion of total costs than in any other field of higher education. Furthermore, graduate students as house staff pay nothing toward their education—in fact, they earn a living wage. Not so for graduate students in nursing and allied health.

Furthermore, by paying salaries to residents, hospitals are in fact directly subsidizing undergraduate medical education, since residents spend 10-15 percent of their time teaching undergraduate MD students.

A number of economists, until recently, believed that the degree of subsidization of medical students was excessive in relation to other fields and to the future earnings potential of physicians.

Distributive Inequity

When support is provided through patient care revenues, inequities result in the distribution of costs, as follows: (1) The elderly whose care is paid for by Medicare use hospitals more than younger population groups. Part A of Medicare is financed through a regressive tax which falls more heavily on low income groups. Part B is somewhat more progressive because premiums are matched by federal general revenues. Costs of education add to the costs of patient care. (2) Private health insurance premiums vary by the size of the group and the experience of the group. High risk industry, employers with older or sicker employees, small companies, and individuals pay higher health insurance premiums than large companies and young, white-collar groups. Again regressive financing; again education costs add to the problem. (3) Teaching hospitals are not distributed proportionate to population. Historically, a larger proportion of teaching hospitals and residencies have been located in the northeastern and midwestern industrial states. Nursing educa tion is more evenly distributed. The health insurance premiums in states with large education programs are subsidizing the training of health professionals who migrate to the sunbelt.

The Escalating Cost of Health Care

Until the Tax Equity and Fiscal Responsibility Act of 1982 and the 1983 Social Security Amendments, except in the few states with rate regulation, hospital payments were essentially open ended. I need not mention the inflation in health care costs. The main point is that there were no restraints on hospital spending in any area. If hospitals wished to expand their education programs, particularly in medicine, the costs were passed through to third-party payers, as reflected in both the hospital costs and charges to patients.

Furthermore, although data are insufficient to prove the assertion, most policy analysts believe that education programs, particularly for MDs, induce more services, particularly ancillary services, and longer lengths of stay, which add further to cost escalation.

Despite the recent changes in reimbursement, Medicare continues to pass through the direct and indirect costs of education, but these provisions are viewed as temporary.

Distortions in Training

Third-party reimbursement for hospital care pays for more than 90 percent of all care in hospitals. Out-of-hospital services are less well covered for the reasons that fewer services are covered by third parties and the patient is responsible for more cost sharing for outpatient services than inpatient services. The result is far more difficulty in generating education support for out-of-hospital training than for training in the hospital. Medicine has relied more heavily on hospital training than has nursing.

Furthermore, the financing agencies have placed no limitations on numbers of students, type of students, or specialty in inpatient settings. The consequences are a heavy support for inpatient training in all fields, but most notably in medicine. HMOs, visiting nurse services, community health centers, and home health agencies cannot easily pass through education costs to consumers.

CURRENT AND POTENTIAL CHANGES IN SUPPORT FOR HEALTH PROFESSIONS EDUCATION

The federal government has terminated, or reduced, a number of programs that provided capitation or project grant support for health professions education. In addition, reductions have been made in student support, with shifts from scholarships to loans and from subsidized to nonsubsidized loans. These changes are the result of policy conclusions that the shortage of health professionals has disappeared and that health professions education should be treated in the same manner as all higher education. The change in loan and scholarship policies reflects both a change in the political orientation of the executive branch of government and the Senate and the high incomes of physicians.

While federal suport for nursing education has fared better than for education of the other health professions due to congressional intervention, a downward trend in nursing education support can be anticipated.

A number of states have begun to cut back support as well, most notably in dental education and now in medical education. Cutbacks in all fields can be anticipated for the following reasons: the perceived consequence of perceived surpluses; the changing demography, for as the baby boom population reaches maturity, the college-age population is declining; and the high cost of the health professions education and competition for funds for other higher education programs, e.g., improved primary and secondary education and other social purposes.

A number of factors have begun to affect the other streams of financial support. Although Congress reversed the President's request for no increase in biomedical research funding in the FY 1984 budget, biomedical research funding had declined in the fiscal years immediately preceding FY 1984. The federal deficit makes unlikely substantial increases in biomedical research funds for the next several years. With the nursing profession just beginning to develop doctoral programs and research bases, the competition from other professions with established research bases places nursing at a disadvantage for this source of funding, unless a special grant program for nursing research is enacted.

The most dramatic changes in support, however, will come from the patient care side, in the following ways.

The development of competition in the health field has spawned several major changes that can affect support for education. Preferred provider organizations (PPOs) are developing which negotiate with hospitals for fixed prices and discounts. Teaching hospitals are at a disadvantage if the decision for a PPO is made on price alone. Hospitals with teaching programs will attempt to pare their costs to compete, and many hospitals have begun to review the scope and size of their education programs.

As HMOs spread, a similar phenomenon can be anticipated. While the Kaiser hospitals have some training programs, most other HMOs do not operate their own hospitals and do not support training programs. If affiliation with teaching hospitals inhibits HMOs from competitive pricing, they will seek arrangements with nonteaching hospitals.

While Medicare has allowed a pass through of direct teaching costs and indirect costs based on resident-to-bed ratios, this is probably a temporary provision. For nursing, the Medicare formula allows pass through of the direct costs, but these costs do not include payment of any portion of the salaries of full-time academic nursing school faculty. No indirect costs for nursing education programs are recognized.

The Social Security Advisory Council has recently recommended that alternatives to patient care support of education costs be explored.

The new Medicare payment system by diagnosis (DRGs) will have indirect effects on the size of the education program in hospitals and the education process itself. For example, if, as conjectured by many, education programs add to the number of tests and procedures per stay and to the lengths of stay, hospitals will try to reduce these additional costs. DRG reimbursement places incentives on doing less and shorter stays. Furthermore, there are incentives to provide services out of the hospital, wherever possible. National data show a decline in admissions and inpatient surgical procedures. Obviously, this trend reduces the clinical base in hospitals for education. There is no evidence that the training programs are moving into HMOs, surgicenters, urgent care centers, etc. This trend will also increase competition among the professions for clinical experience. Just visualize a university hospital or the principal teaching hospital for an academic health center with declining admissions and a declining patient base. Who will have priority in education—medicine, pharmacy, nursing?

The concern over maldistribution of the specialties in medicine has led some commentators to suggest setting numerical limits or dollar limits on support of residency programs. Some have suggested eliminating patient care support and making direct grants for education support. Others believe that the sick, the low income, and the elderly should not bear disproportionate costs of health professions education. States which are exporters of manpower are also questioning whether their citizens should pay for training of professionals who move elsewhere.

In the next five years, growing pressures can be expected to reduce support for education and particularly to reduce support from patient care funds. These pressures will come from two directions. First, increased competition and changes in reimbursement will force reevaluation of the size and costs of education programs. Second, policy debates will propose changing patient care support or limiting support by the following options:

- Shifting from third-party payments to direct grants from states or the federal government with control on total numbers of students;

- Taxing all public and private payers a percentage amount to provide direct grants for education;

- Placing a ceiling on the amount Medicare will pay, which will be quickly followed by Medicaid and other third parties;

- Expecting the students to bear more of the costs through tuition.

While these prospects may seem gloomy, nursing will be less affected than medicine because it has had to rely much more on state support, contributed costs of voluntary agencies other than hospitals, and tuition. Furthermore, because nursing did not have as open ended or lavish support as medicine, nursing has been far more cost conscious and cost effective in its training programs. As the economy improves, there may again be a shortage of nurses and hospitals may see advantages to continuing their involvement in nursing education.

The dangers for nursing will come from other external factors, including the increasing competition between physicians and other professions, particularly nurse practitioners, for jobs and caseloads for clinical training, both within and outside of hospitals.

THE IMPACT OF DRGs ON EDUCATIONAL PROGRAMS IN NURSING

Sara E. Smith

Reviewing the changes that created the climate which produced DRGs gives a frame of reference to better understand the total picture. For me, at least, it is impossible to consider the implications of DRGs for nursing education in isolation from other societal changes.

John Naisbitt, in his best-seller *Megatrends,* has identified ten trends he believes are shaping the future. All of what he says is applicable to health care, some trends more directly than others. The four that seem most directly related to nursing are: the move from an industrial to an information society; the high-tech/high-touch age; the change from the either/or option to multiple options; and the trend from institutional help to self-help.

Naisbitt, a news analyst, draws heavily on Toffler's predictions. In his latest book, *Previews and Premises,* Toffler applies Nobel Prize-winner Ilya Prigogine's work on the thermodynamics of nonequilibrium systems to the changes going on in our world. Prigogine has said that any phenomenon, a chemical compound or a social system, is always undergoing internal change, always fluctuating. Each system or phenomenon has its own internal subsystems, each of which is also vibrating or fluctuating. Occasionally, one of these fluctuations becomes so intense that the subsystem shatters. More commonly, several subsystems converge and reinforce one another to alter or revolutionize the main system substantially. Each system or phenomenon has an external environment where fluctuations occur as well. If a large external fluctuation coincides with the conjuncture of several internal fluctuations, a revolutionary change or transformation may occur.[1]

We are witnessing this revolution in the health care system. What will be the shape of this transformation or revolutionary change? I certainly don't have

---

[1] Alvin Toffler, *Reviews and Premises* (New York: William Morrow & Co., 1983), p. 172.

the answers, but I do have a lot of questions, and I am going to suggest some possibilities. I am confident that each reader will think of other possibilities.

Are DRGs a crisis or a challenge? I see them as a challenge with a multitude of exciting opportunities for health care and particularly the nursing profession. (Of course, one of my colleagues continually tells me I am a Pollyanna.) To explain my point of view, I have grouped my comments into three general areas: curriculum and planned learning experiences, cost and financial factors, and ethical considerations. Since the three interrelate and overlap, the same or similar factors may be mentioned more than once.

CURRICULUM AND PLANNED LEARNING EXPERIENCES

One of the predictable outcomes of the implementation of the DRG system will be shorter patient stays and thus more rapid turnover, with the result of fewer patients in the hospital at any one time. Reduced census is always difficult for the nurse educator who attempts to find sufficient assignments for students without overloading an area with students. However, the reduced number of patients in the future will probably be more acutely ill. In the past three or four years, even before the advent of DRGs, it had become increasingly difficult to find suitable patient assignments for beginning students. One can only anticipate that once DRGs are fully implemented, appropriate assignments for beginning students may be impossible without rethinking our current system. Will it be necessary to give students more practice in the laboratory, a system some educators have never believed was good? My own school has used an extended care facility for several years for students' initial experience; the focus is on skills, and we have found it to be an excellent experience. Even so, the transition to the acute-care system is difficult for students. Another option for the initial experience would be nursing homes. Will the traditional ratio of 8-12 students to each instructor in the acute-care setting have to be altered to 4-6 students for each instructor as students master basic skills with acutely ill patients with complex illnesses? If so, will students be willing or able to pay what this type of education may cost?

Reduced census also dictates that faculty evaluate carefully the number of students admitted to the program each year. If a 600-bed facility which has adequately accommodated a student population of 200 cuts back its average patient census to 500, is a parallel reduction in student population required? We may be fooling ourselves if we continue to believe the census problem is only a temporary phenomenon.

A more complex question in number of admissions is how to predict what the job market will be like for new graduates in three or four years. We recognize that the marketplace is changing and the demand for nurses has leveled off except in a few areas throughout the United States. If we believe this trend will remain the same or perhaps accelerate under the DRG system, we have an obligation to at least consider accepting fewer students. We certainly do not want to graduate the same numbers we did during the nurse shortage of the sixties and seventies.

Should curricula change to prepare the nurse of the future? The answer is a resounding yes. Although my list is not all-inclusive, I have developed eight points to consider in this regard:

1. Our rapidly growing elderly population, the group that first felt the impact of DRGs, continues to provide unique challenges. The curriculum must address the process of aging with at least the same emphasis that is given to growth and development. Nutrition, medications, home care, community agencies, and volunteer groups are a few of the suggestions that come to mind.

   We need to do a better job of teaching students the rewards of working with the elderly and to reinforce the need for highly skilled, competent RNs to work in nursing homes and extended-care facilities. These facilities will care for many of the patients who face earlier discharge from the hospital under the DRG system.

2. The late seventies and early eighties have seen Americans turn to wellness and assume responsibility for maintaining their own health. Although nursing has long held wellness and health as a goal, we have only recently begun to teach students about wellness. It is hard to let go of the medical model and the disease process as the focus of the curriculum, perhaps because the disease process is clearly defined and learning pathophysiology yields a sense of accomplishment, whereas the profession is just beginning to develop nursing theory. We are still in the early stages of documenting the difference between nursing and medicine. We all know nursing is different from medicine, but the differences become elusive when we try to base a curriculum on the nursing model. If we believe that health or wellness is more than just the absence of disease, we must begin to focus on just that and teach our students how to make healthy people healthier. What profession is better suited to being in the pivotal position during this transitional era in health care? The opportunity is present for health care to become truly *health care,* rather than illness care.

3. The report from the Institute of Medicine indicated that two-thirds of the 1.3 million nurses employed in 1980 worked in the nation's hospitals.[2] As the number of hospital beds in use throughout the nation decreases, so will the need for registered nurses in the acute-care setting. The hospitalized patient will be more acutely ill and require a nurse highly skilled in technical skills, so it may be that more registered nurses will be needed to care for fewer patients; but I think it reasonable to assume that hospitals will not continue to need two-thirds of all the nation's

---

[2] *Nursing and Nursing Education: Public Policies and Private Actions* (Washington, DC: National Academy Press, 1983), p. 1.

nurses. We need to reconsider home health care and other alternatives to the acute-care setting. Opportunity abounds for nursing practice in uncharted areas, and we can create the parameters of these new areas.

4. Frank Shaffer states that the "nursing department must become responsible for educating the patient and his family at the time of admission concerning expected length of stay and discharge."[3] Discharge planning takes on a different shape when it is incorporated into the admission process. Communication and coordination of care between hospital and home health care nurses, always important, become essential as patients go home with sophisticated treatment regimens. We must teach students to think about and plan for the home care needs of the patient while the patient is in the acute-care setting. Even though we have always done some of this, it is a different ballgame now with about three fewer innings to win the game. The student will need a better knowledge of the available community resources so as to teach a patient how to take maximum advantage of those resources. More and more, the nurse will be responsible for coordination of care, teaching, and follow-up care. As I think of all the new graduate is expected to know, my head spins! Yet we must lay the foundation in undergraduate study if the graduate is to function as a professional.

5. John Naisbitt believes that we "mass-produce information the way we used to mass-produce cars" and that "the new source of power is not money in the hands of a few but information in the hands of many."[4]

   One of the ways to manage the tremendous volume of available information is through the use of computers. Computers can create order out of the chaos of too much data. Our students must appreciate the role that computers and information systems will play in nursing. Awareness could be developed in a variety of ways, from computer-assisted instruction throughout the nursing program to a computer literacy course in the curriculum. So much of what our world is today results directly from our computer society. And it should be remembered that the development of the DRG system of reimbursement was possible only through the use of computers.

   Programs are already available that list appropriate nursing interventions once sufficient data on the patient has been entered into the computer. Increasingly sophisticated programs may drastically alter what we teach in the classroom. I wonder how much we teach because it has always been taught or because the students might need to know it. Perhaps we are like the sages in Peddiwell's *Saber-Tooth Curriculum* who valued a curriculum for its timelessness, rather than its timeliness.[5]

---

[3] Franklin A. Shaffer, "Nursing: Gearing Up for DRGs, Part II: Management Strategies," *Nursing & Health Care*, 5:2:98, February 1984.

[4] John Naisbitt, *Megatrends* (New York: Warner Books, Inc., 1982), p. 16.

[5] J. Abner Peddiwell, *The Saber-Toothed Curriculum* (New York: McGraw-Hill Book Company, 1939), pp. 24-44.

6. Perhaps the DRG system offers nursing unique opportunities because of the changes it is creating in health care. Nurses spend a great deal of time creating, collecting, and disseminating information through teaching, speaking, counseling, and research for patients or clients and society as a whole. We are contributing to the information society, but I am not sure we always recognize that valuable service. Just as it is essential for the student to learn pathophysiology and the nursing process, she/he must also acquire an awareness of what a nurse will contribute to the information society. The nurse has a powerful position in this new information society. Who else is better suited to assist society in adjusting to the new health care of the eighties, help an individual evaluate his options and make the best choice, teach an individual how to be more responsible for his health, and provide an individual with the information he needs? I admit to a bias, but I don't think anyone is better suited than the professional nurse.

7. In addition to what we have previously considered essential for any nursing curriculum, we need to consider educating a nurse who is "businesswise" and has knowledge of efficient utilization of human resources and organizational strategy. Is this appropriate to an undergraduate curriculum? The new graduate does not function in a management position as a head nurse or supervisor; however, she does function in an organizational hierarchy, if only to manage two or three workers in primary care or five or six members of a team. Basic knowledge about working with groups and especially about the process of decision making, both individually and as a group, will aid the nurse. Perhaps this is already taught and we need not concern ourselves with it; or perhaps a faculty group will decide it is not appropriate for their particular curriculum. However, I believe the nurse of the eighties and beyond will find it essential.

8. The DRG system will force us to articulate clearly what nursing is and what nursing is not. If we do not, nursing may face extinction. Most nurses can easily identify a personal belief about what nursing is, yet we continue to allow others, be they doctors or administrators, to impose their view of nursing upon us. As competition increases for a piece of the health care dollar, it becomes urgent for us to say how nursing makes a difference, and not to allow valuable nursing experience to be wasted on non-nursing tasks. We need to be assertive about the identity of the nurse. We must also do a better job of instilling in our students a sense of responsibility for supporting community activities as well as contributing to local, state, and national policy forums and health care planning groups. Who is better prepared to make recommendations or decisions about health care than nurses? Nursing must represent its own interests in the political arena and must educate the politicians and public alike to what nursing is and what it is not.

Our students need to feel competent and to know they possess the basic knowledge to make good decisions and, equally important, they need the ability to utilize a variety of resources to find an answer or solve a problem.

COST AND FINANCIAL FACTORS

We have heard a variety of predictions about the disastrous change we can expect in health care as a result of the implementation of DRGs. Some reports filtering in indicate that hospitals may be able to show a profit under the DRG system. It will be some time before the final verdict is in; however, some things are predictable and they include the following:

1. An article in the January 1984 issue of *Trustee,* the magazine for hospital governing boards, points out that the most significant change among boards of directors in New Jersey since DRGs were introduced three years ago "has been more aggressive questioning by trustees about whether hospital programs should be cut."[6] There is a need to identify "winners and losers"—programs that are financially viable and those that are not.

2. Many authorities suggest that hospitals may begin to market services, especially to businesses. Could nurse educators be creative and innovative in marketing nursing services to the community and business? Businesses will be looking for less expensive ways to provide fringe benefits for employees. Would they be willing to pay for an informational health service provided by nurses? We need to examine the marketplace to determine if nursing is offering what the consumers want, need, or will buy. We would have to be blind not to recogize that Americans are very interested in becoming healthier. Just browse through any popular magazine; each one will have at least one article on health. How many are written by nurses? Yet most nurses identify the goal of nursing as health. Consumers seek information about health in those places where it is most readily available. A classmate of mine has never practiced nursing in the traditional sense; yet she has operated a highly successful health spa in Atlanta for several years. She readily admits that she frequently utilizes her nursing knowledge in counseling clients about diet, exercise, and health habits. Her authority for counseling is to say, "Of course I know about these things; I am a nurse." Another friend and classmate worked in a diet client in New York City to support herself while studying for a doctorate. She too relies on her nursing background as she counsels clients. In both situations, clients pay substantial fees for these services; clients probably would not identify nursing as the service they are purchasing but, in fact, it is.

---

[6]Charles M. Ewell, "A Look at How New Jersey's DRG System Is Changing Board Role," *Trustee,* 37:28, January 1984.

Is it possible for faculty to develop a clinic or home health agency staffed partially by faculty and utilized for student experiences? I believe we have to rethink the boundaries of the practice of nursing. I know we are on the brink of change, and it can be a marvelous opportunity for us.

Education continues to be a pass-through cost under the DRG system, but for how long is anybody's guess. Most people who are willing to speculate don't expect any change during the phase-in period or for the first few years beyond. Increasingly, the question is asked: Should the sick and injured bear the cost of medical education? In reality, under Medicare, we taxpayers pay the greatest share of those costs through our contributions to Social Security.

The report of the Institute of Medicine included the recommendation that "institutional and student financial support should be maintained by state and local governments, higher education institutions, hospitals, and third-party payers to assure that generalist nursing education programs have capacity and enrollments sufficient to graduate the numbers and kinds of nurses commensurate with state and local goals for the nurse supply."[7] The National Commission on Nursing made a similar recommendation. So there are those who advocate continued financial support of nursing education; we have to wonder, though, with the current shortage of nursing positions, if this will change.

ETHICAL CONSIDERATIONS

Without a crystal ball, I am not sure what ethical considerations will arise, especially considerations specific to nursing education. We can be sure that hospitals will encourage or even seek out the profitable DRG admissions, which creates concern about who will care for the unprofitable ones. We may begin to see a very different balance of types or categories of patients. Student clinical experiences will be affected by this, but if we are truly teaching conceptually and not depending on disease conditions, perhaps it won't matter.

There is some speculation that physicians may play an even greater role in hospitals in decisions related to service provision, resource allocation, and staffing. If this is true, then nurses must seek a greater role as well. Educators cannot afford to sit by and expect nursing service colleagues to be responsible for the changes. The collective voice of nursing should be heard.

Concern for cost threatens to exceed concern for improving quality; yet quality need not depend solely on cost. We can expect that hospitals will increasingly specialize in what they do well, both clinically and economically. Quality, it can then be posited, will thus be sustained and perhaps even enhanced. Difficult decisions are projected for the future. Will there be two levels of care? Will someone be denied admission to a hospital for transplant surgery because of inadequate insurance? Will patients actually be turned out in the street when their insurance runs out? We could think of endless questions, but only speculate about the answers. What we can do is have a voice

---

[7]*Nursing and Nursing Education, op. cit.,* p. 5.

in the decision-making process, through our place of employment, through our local community, and through local, state, and national government. If there are fewer health care dollars, nurses owe it to students, patients, and community to see that those health care dollars are wisely spent.

DRGs are here; our choice is how we will deal with them. We can choose to be resigned and react to circumstances, or we can choose to be optimistic and look for opportunities.

THE EFFECTS OF PROSPECTIVE REIMBURSEMENT ON NURSING EDUCATION

Susan C. Reinhard

This much is clear about prospective reimbursement: the external forces of regulatory controls on financing health care will induce changes throughout the health care delivery system. We have seen several generations of regulations in health care: institutional budget caps, Health Systems Agencies, Professional Standards Review Organizations, and the like. Attempts to control health care access, quality, and cost have come mainly through planning and regulation of the *settings* of health care—particularly hospitals since they ring up the largest health care bill. However, control of the hospital budget through administrative controls and budget caps has been unsuccessful because administrators are not the ones who really run up the bill; the *providers* do. It makes sense, then, that true reform of the system could not take place until there was institutional control of the provider through cost control of ordering practices. This is what prospective rate setting is all about. It is an external effort to curb costs by limiting resource use by the providers according to logical guidelines established in the DRG predictions of what homogeneous groups of clients should require.

Our challenge is to project the probable scope and potential impact of this mechanism of external regulatory control on nursing practice, administration, and education. We *will* adapt in some way, because we are an essential part of the health care system and because we will be forced to do so. What we must do is anticipate the requirements of the new system so that we can form our role in it *proactively*—that is, before that role is dictated by others.

This paper is intended to explore the ramifications of the fiscal realities and political/regulatory climate on nursing education: what is happening now and what we need to do to whip ourselves into shape in terms of our curricula for basic and advanced preparation for practice, our political sophistication, and our research emphasis.

Prospective-reimbursement mechanisms imposed by governmental regulations will alter incentive structures and reshape behavioral relationships among providers in settings that adopt this financial reform tool. These phenomena are already occurring in New Jersey hospitals, which have used this system for four years. We will probably also find ourselves facing DRGs in other health care delivery settings, such as skilled nursing facilities and home health. The Health Care Financing Administration (HCFA) has been working on a draft proposal for long-term facilities, which should be ready by June 1984; the draft proposals for home health care will probably be available by June 1985. By then, the whole health care delivery system will be grappling with DRGs or some kind of case-mix prospective rate-setting mechanism. Therefore, we can anticipate that most, if not all of the graduates of our nursing programs will experience first-hand fundamental changes in practice delivery. A new kind of "teamwork" is evolving with the potential for an increased power base for graduates who are prepared to steer the ship. We have to teach what the market demands and what the profession must do to control its destiny.

EDUCATION FOR A NEW ERA

New Skills in the Marketplace

What new skills will our students require to accomplish these objectives? The skills are not new, but are more sophisticated and more critical for survival than before. I would like to focus on five major areas: the accessing and creation of data, communication and collaboration, clinical and management practice, fiscal accountability, and political savvy.

At all levels, the most obvious need is the development of computer and statistical skills. The prospective rate-setting methodology is data intensive; that is, it requires an enormous amount of regulatory information. A number of different personnel can provide, code, and report these data. The critical point is that nurses who are comfortable with computers can *use* these sophisticated data, which combine the financial and clinical dimensions of client care. They can use this information to build their case for nursing—for the integrity of the nursing budget, for protection of the staff size and skill mix, and for a rationale for the cost effectiveness of their mode of care delivery. Nurses interested in continuing primary nursing in their hospitals will have to document its money-saving features. The quality dimension of care will have to be documented in cold, hard facts that can be translated into computer-manipulated figures. Unless we can *market* quality in language the system understands, it will be deaf to our pleas for improved care alternatives. All nurses will be expected to be able to participate in sophisticated data processing; if they cannot, other personnel will replace them or at least take over essential nursing information-gathering functions. Therefore, courses in statistics, computer use, and marketing will become necessities in the curriculum.

A second set of skills necessary for our graduates to survive in a DRG world involves communication and collaboration. We have long been strong in the area of interpersonal communications. Our students and graduates are highly skilled in this domain when communication is centered on nurse-client exchanges. *This will not be enough.* We must prepare our students for the *business* of nursing and the communications strategies that business demands.

We have recognized that nurses cannot tolerate the transactional neurosis inherent in the well-known "nurse-physician game." We cannot afford such nonsense in this corporate environment. Teachers must be attuned to students' communication patterns with other providers as closely as they are to student-client interactions. Students need to role-play and to practice effective colleague communication patterns. Direct observation or at least filmed examination of verbal and non-verbal communication strategies utilized in interdisciplinary management meetings would be helpful. We already know how to teach communication; what we need is to redirect our focus to accommodate anticipated system changes.

A third set of skills, which we already teach but need to refocus, include those in nursing practice responsibilities, both clinical and management.

Emphasis on disease prevention and health promotion is congruent with the cost-conscious climate as well as nursing's philosophy. During a luncheon at the N.J. League for Nursing Convention in April 1984, Senator Bill Bradley of New Jersey arrived at some important conclusions about the emerging model of health care delivery in the U.S. as a result of health cost-consciousness in our society. This new model of health care delivery more closely resembles the nursing model of health care: (1) there is a focus on prevention, to keep people out of hospitals; (2) there is an emphasis on the individual's responsibility for health care; and (3) there is a shift to non-institutionalization.

Seem familiar? Seems to me like things that nurses have been pushing for many years, things that we are uniquely able to do! But now we'll have some external forces on our side: for example, people will be rewarded for taking charge of their own health through the lower rates offered by insurance companies to those who keep their weight down, stop smoking, and buckle up in the car. The assumption is that *money talks*, and as behaviorists say, people will behave in ways which are positively rewarded. These are lifestyle changes that require health teaching, and this is the area in which nurses can shine! Unfortunately, up to now, the patient education focus has been largely directed toward the management of illness rather than toward its prevention. Prevention has not been a priority because there was what Lucille Joel calls a "blank-check mentality" to treating disease. Now, however, that pay-as-you-exit check has been changed to a pay-as-you-enter price tag, and third-party reimbursers are seeking ways to prevent that entrance altogether. Nursing is the profession most ready for this new wave. We must teach our students to seize this opportunity by showing them how to market these skills, get third-party reimbursement, and set up nurse-run clinics as well as private practices. They will find that reimbursement opportunities will exist, but only if they can present the data to document their ability to do more for the money than other providers.

Competition is the password. Research is the key. Legislation will be the process. We have just obtained third-party reimbursement for nurses in New Jersey through legislative changes in the Blue Shield provider regulations. We must all do what we can to get the Community Nursing Centers bill through Congress. Tom Nickels, the ANA Washington lobbyist, has told me that any legislation we get through to establish independent, nurse-run clinics will also include prospective rate-setting as part of the package. So we will have to get ourselves and our students prepared for DRGs in our own settings as well—for both illness care and wellness teaching.

Community health experiences: The case mix in the community will become more complex and acute due to earlier hospital discharge. Students should be encouraged to explore their potential roles in the home, where nursing has always been strong. With the trend to home health gathering momentum and reimbursement, all providers are turning attention to this domain. New physicians may indeed return to house-call practice if that is where clients are to be found in this competitive health market. Community Medicaid waiver programs for home care in six of the seven N.J. counties eligible are being managed by social workers. We should remind our students of our rich history in the home and our rightful place in supervising and directing policies related to home health care. Teach them that they must prove their worth in this setting as well as in the hospital.

Early discharge planning is a related concept. The new system demands discharge planning from the moment of admission, and our graduates will be expected to perform in this mode. They will be held accountable for initiating and monitoring the plan. And they should bear in mind that any increase in length of stay that can be traced to nursing's being remiss will be charged to nursing in some form—from reprimand to dismissal of erring nurses. The concept of trim points should be introduced to students, and some actual experience with utilization review and discharge planning must be incorporated into the curriculum.

Observational skills must be sharpened. Assessments must be immediate and thorough. We can't rely on technology. We need to go back to our earlier skills of watching the client for early signs of complications so that prompt attention can be given without an undue increase in length of stay. We have to teach our students sophisticated nursing—to develop a keen eye, to trust their observations and assessments, and to act on them responsibly. Those who wait for the physician or technology to intervene will eventually find themselves out of a job. Although students may want to focus on the "doctorly" skills of auscultation and assessment of heart murmurs and not on measuring edema, the real nurse's image stresses the basics and demands sensitive observations and measurements.

Coordination skills will be demanded of nurses. We will be expected to set the therapeutic plan in motion and keep the momentum going smoothly to accomplish discharge on time. We have always taught this role to students.

We have to highlight clinical experiences for developing such coordinating skills. Computer-game simulations dealing with coordination would be of enormous value. Students could work through decision trees to practice the efficiency as well as the quality of their clinical judgments in patient care. Other items that require nurses' skill in coordination are: juggling client scheduling for tests and procedures, meals, personal care, as well as stop orders and preps for procedures.

Documentation of observation will be critical. Everything will have to be documented precisely and concisely. Our students must learn early that we did what we write that we did, not what we say we did. Reimbursement will address the scope and depth only of the documented care. As we move into sophisticated systems of reimbursement based on nursing resource use, or relative intensity measures (RIMs), we will become increasingly dependent on the quality of documentation, which will translate into the size of the nursing budget.

Students need practice in *writing*. They should be given many opportunities to develop skill in the various forms of writing that will be required of them: nurses' notes, clinical reports, financial reports, memos, and letters. In addition, students should be taught the importance of documenting their observations and practice in such a way as to influence the ordering practices of other providers. As Dr. Lucille Joel has pointed out in the literature, a physician's ordering practices can be curtailed when nurses provide sensitive clinical data in a cogent, reliable manner.[1] Data provided by nurses will also be used to document outliers.

The Challenge of Fiscal Accountability

In addition to these practice dimensions, all students need to be prepared to *assume a role in fiscal accountability*. As future staff nurses, students should be ready to accept individual budgetary responsibility. Our graduates should expect to share the burden of containing costs and providing the data their nurse managers require. Educators must convey a philosophy of cost-consciousness throughout the curriculum, because managing money and resources is now every nurse's concern. If students understand their role, modeled by their instructors and colleagues in clinical practice settings, they will have a greater economic conscience. Medical students at the University of Medicine and Dentistry of New Jersey now take an innovative course to sensitize them to the costs of their ordering practices; topics include financing health care, cost-containment strategies, cost efficiency, competition in health care, and DRGs. Other medical schools believe cost-effectiveness should be a thread woven throughout the curriculum; that is, in every clinical situation, medical students should be taught to ask themselves: What does this cost? Can it be done cheaper without sacrificing quality?

[1]Lucille Joel, "DRGs: The State of the Art of Reimbursement for Nursing Services," *Nursing & Health Care,* 4(10):563, December 1983.

Nursing students must be socialized in the same manner. We need to undo old values. The words and the music have to go together or our students will not integrate this cost-conscious philosophy into their attitudes and behaviors. Values clarification exercises would be enlightening and beneficial—for students and teachers alike. Many of us are products of the blank-check era. We have to become aware of our values and become sensitized to how they influence our behavior in practice. It would also be educational for the student to investigate the "trim points" for clients in specific DRG categories and explore ways to accomplish the goals and objectives of the nursing care plan within that time frame. Methods of saving money on materials and procedures could also be explored in post-conferences. Students need to see an incentive for creatively cutting costs and managing a budget in terms of potential wage increases, increased staff, and the like.

By the same token, we should help shape the students' perceptions of their own monetary value to the institutions in which they work. This is a new concept, a new self-image for nurses who generally see themselves as altruistic providers of services. They need to see themselves as valuable providers of essential services that are worth money, that they are in the business of nursing and that the product is the patient. Students should be indoctrinated in the marketplace values of entrepreneurs; they do not have to be in private practice to have the self-concept of being worth money because of their specialized knowledge and skills. They should have a sense of their ability to generate income—that they aren't just "costs."

At the same time that we socialize our students into cost-consciousness and their economic value, it is imperative that we continue to emphasize nursing's social contract with the client. Yes, we must be penny-wise and monetarily sophisticated, but the professions must remain the guardians of quality of care. The student should learn from the beginning of the education/socialization process that a nurse is an autonomous professional whose practice decisions cannot be based solely on data from the financial officer.

The Politics of Economics

Finally, to deal with the larger picture, students should be prepared to understand the economics of health care delivery and how these dynamics impact upon their daily practice and future careers. This preparation should begin in freshman—not senior—year in a generalized course focusing on the issues and concepts as well as the "buzz words" inherent in the new system. Obviously, today's students need to know what case-mixed reimbursement is all about and the active role the profession will expect of them in establishing nursing as a reimbursable cost center. However, since no one can predict what regulations will be created in the future, our students need to know regulatory history and process, as well as their potential role in formulating policies that will define their practice. Some regulatory mechanism will always exist and will therefore have an impact on nursing. We will need politically astute and active graduates who will attain elected and appointed positions of regulatory power so that the voice of nursing will be heard. We need politically astute and active graduates who know that policy is formulated through compromise and pressure and can take many years to develop (like third-party reimbursement) or can happen so quickly it makes you dizzy (like the prospective payment legislation, which took only three months).

Help your students set their goals high. We need nurses in appointed offices: on regulatory boards, in the departments of health, on hospital boards of trustees, and on the boards of all kinds of health agencies—wherever decisions are made. We also need them as elected lawmakers at all levels of government.

How do we shape such nursing political gladiators? By teaching them from the first year that their political involvement is necessary because (1) their license to practice comes through law; (2) the right to practice in general, specialized, and expanded roles is influenced by law; and (3) their workplaces are governed by laws and regulations, which in turn affect them.

Show students how to get involved:

- Connect politics with practice issues
- Have them debate the issues in class or conferences
- Require them to write a letter to a legislator about something that concerns them
- Work through student organizations to sponsor a trip to the capital or state house
- Invite a legislator to come and talk to students.

Be creative—the point is to demystify politics through practice.

Beyond the legislative and regulatory arenas, students need to become sensitive to the politics of power, authority, and change within health care institutions. If they are to claim a piece of the pie, they have to know how to slice it! Invite experienced nurse administrators to address your students; there is no substitute for a strong role model.

Graduate Education

What I have discussed thus far can be applied to all levels of nursing education. But what about the preparation of our leaders in advanced practice, teaching, and administration? Our graduate programs in nursing will need revisions in the internal curriculum and external marketing approach for recruitment of students. Graduate education has evolved in the past due to changes in societal and student needs. We are now challenged to adapt again.

Graduate programs began with the goal of generalized advanced preparation for students who largely sought employment in the nursing education sector, and later in nursing administration. However, technology grew and new, competing providers emerged to fill the public's need for the primary and specialized care that the depressed supply of physicians could not provide. Our graduate schools shifted gears and began to prepare clinical specialists with in-depth knowledge of clusters of phenomena, physical assessment skills, and knowledge of nursing theory and research. Graduates were advised to enter the health care market and "sell themselves," create their own job descriptions, and broaden the boundaries of the nursing role. Students who entered these programs shared this vision and challenge. They believed they could forge new clinical specialist and practitioner roles within the expansive climate of health policy and funding that existed after the enactment of Medicare and Medicaid. Many have succeeded, and those who participated in their preparation should take pride in knowing they were well prepared.

The problem we face now is a new climate—one that is cool toward the development of any provider role which cannot demonstrate its cost-effectiveness. There are new rules to the game and new skills necessary in order to win. Prospective graduate students seem to be questioning the vision and promise of our graduate programs; they are not convinced either that we can prepare them for the responsibilities they will be required to assume or that there will be jobs for them upon completion of our rigorous programs.

Administration. Why are prospective students of nursing admministration so skeptical of the value of the MSN? They are wary of nursing's ability to provide them with the level of sophistication in finance that they foresee as being essential. Some are opting for an MBA in addition to, or instead of, their MSN. They claim that the nursing administration minor is "good for getting your feet wet, but not enough for talking with the big boys."

These students are torn. They recognize that turning toward another discipline for graduate work may retard the growth of the knowledge base in nursing theory and research. Indeed, by opting for an MBA instead of an MSN, they are in effect closing the door on potential future careers in education. However, they are perceptive and they are realists. Since power bases are shifting, with the finance officer assuming a greater share of the power, future nurse administrators will need to speak in the same tongue so they can be heard.

Perhaps we need to consider graduate academic articulation with colleges of management and finance just as we have sought in the past similar meeting grounds with colleges of medicine for physical assessment. They may be a temporary arrangement until we have developed enough nursing faculty experts in these fields to offer truly distinct courses. But if we don't do something, we risk losing our future brightest nurse managers to other fields of study. We cannot stand idle and witness such a brain drain.

Clinical specialists. We may also need to rethink our philosophy of graduate education of clinical specialists. Institutions operating in a prospective-payment, cost-containment world are looking for ways to cut down. Clinical specialists who cannot prove their worth in dollars and cents, as well as in quality of care, will be the first to go. The powers-that-be at the upper levels of decision making must view clinical specialists as something more than "super staff nurses." These specialists can and should be a "differentiating variable" for health care institutions; that is, they should attract clients because thet can provide a level of care unavailable at competing institutions.

How can we teach our clinical specialist students how to prove their worth? In addition to knowing how to read reports and understand computers, they will need to create data that document that their services are what the consumer needs and wants and that they are cost-effective to institutions and to society. For instance, how does their expertise in pain control translate into increased quality of care, decreased length of stay, decreased nursing resource consumption, decreased use of ancillary services and products? Is there a decline in the need to answer call lights, a decreased need to consult the physician for a change in prescriptions, and a decreased number of analgesics and narcotics administered, an increase in client comfort, an earlier discharge? We know this is possible and that it actually occurs; what we have to do is teach our clinical specialists how to document their actions, translate them into numbers, and take their case to upper management. Therefore, in addition to direct clinical nursing and practice-oriented research, these students must also learn the fiscal realities. They, too, need courses in management and finance; they need to know how to conduct research that will relate nursing practice to cost containment (cost savings produced can then be reclaimed for the nursing budget and the hiring of additional clinical specialists, instead of being recaptured into the general budget and being allocated to all departments). Nurse administrators must support this effort in order not to lose the "quality chips" that set them apart, since patients often select the hospital which has the best nursing reputation.

Teaching. Finally, teaching our teachers will be crucial. We are not all comfortable with computers and management information systems, finance, regulatory processes, and political activism. We need continuing education programs as well as formal courses. Our graduate programs with minors in nursing education will have to incorporate the same general principles of finance, management, policy formation that we expect to teach our students.

Research. In terms of research, our graduate and doctoral programs are already directing nurses to examine practice dimensions. Research in the financial components of practice should be incorporated to increase access by opening up reimbursement based on our cost-effectiveness. Such research would be welcomed by the regulatory community as well. We need to produce the evidence that nursing makes a difference, that what we do influences the resource consumption of clients, that highly sophisticated nursing care and documentation influences other providers' ordering practices and decreases the client's length of stay.

If ever there was time the sick in hospitals needed a strong professional nurse at the bedside, it is now. It's up to us to demonstrate this basic fact of life. If we wish to continue the primary nursing mode of delivery, we will have to prove its worth or we will revert to a team-nursing system. This kind of research into comparative modes, although *directed* from the top by a well-prepared nurse administrator, can be *performed* from the bottom up by staff nurses we have prepared in nursing research.

Nor does research have to be limited to in-house concerns. Community-based research will be increasingly sought as we look for alternatives to institutional care. We should look carefully at exactly what it is we do that the market may be seeking under the present conditions. For instance, we know that control of *chronic disease conditions* is a priority in the community now. We should capitalize on that focus, especially since nurses are so well prepared in this area. Research has shown a positive correlation between the care of nurse practioners and greater client compliance with hypertension control regimens. The next step is to demonstrate how this increased compliance translates into fewer hospital admissions and fewer complications that necessitate costlier levels of care.

EFFECTS ON FUNDING OF NURSING EDUCATION

What about the direct effects of prospective rate setting on the educational system and clinical placements? Reimbursement to hospitals for educational costs is in jeopardy. The federal focus now is on medical education; but what happens in this arena will have a ripple effect on nursing education. There is at present an additional reimbursement line for teaching hospitals, but the federal government wants to cut off this pass-through. Who, then, will bear the cost of clinical education? Lobbyists from the New Jersey Hospital Association claim that colleges will be billed for clinical experiences and use of facilities.

Nursing should start thinking of a possible whiplash from this issue. We should begin to validate our contributions to the institutions in which we place our students. We should think in terms of *corporate ventures* and be prepared to answer the institution's question, "What are you going to do for me if I let your students use my valuable and shrinking resources?" Cost it out now for bargaining later. Some schools are providing inservice education or orientation for the hospital; perhaps such internal transfers of services rather than monies are the answer for the present. The financial bargaining process is fundamentally different from the apprentice-service model of education because the separation between educational and service institutions and purposes remains. Cost-benefit analysis of the relationship is a simple marketing technique in an increasingly market-oriented environment.

Another corporate-type venture might be the establishment by educational institutions of clinics for health teaching. Revenues could be returned to education. At the same time, faculty could be actively engaged in practice and maintaining their clinical and management skills in a "real world" environment.

OTHER SOURCES FOR TEACHING DRGs

Continuing Education

There are more and more continuing education programs addressing DRGs, so I believe nurse leaders are learning the ropes of this new game. Unfortunately

I usually don't see too many staff nurses at such programs. Somehow the topic seems to be more interesting to teachers and managers than to staff nurses, who seem to feel DRGs are not their problem yet.

Inservice Education

Perhaps what we need, to drive this subject home to staff nurses, is more inservice education. Some hospitals have been doing inservice on DRGs and RIMs for several years now; these are offered periodically as one-hour programs to keep the staff informed. However, these are in the hospitals that already have DRG experts as nursing directors. Other hospital directors and inservice educators I've talked with say they've done ''a little,'' but that other practice problems have to take priority. The low priority for DRGs and RIMs is probably due to budgets that are so constrained that they can only afford the bare bones of maintaining quality skill levels and introducing new equipment techniques.

Orientation Programs

A hospital's orientation program is another likely placement for DRG education. Yet hospitals that are trying to stay out of the red will be cutting the ''fluff'' out of their budgets, and orientation programs may be one of the first targets. One wonders how much longer they will be able to provide twelve weeks of orientation to our new graduates.

Some hospital administrators are already balking and asking why they can't get a more clinically experienced graduate from our schools. They are asking why they should bear the cost of what we failed to provide. On the other hand, businesses orient their people, and then give them a raise!

This is a serious concern and controversy. Just when the demands on our graduates' clinical skills are the greatest, institutional support for refining those skills may be reduced.

This, too, may be a fertile field for bargaining between education and service.

SUMMARY

In summary, while we educate nurses to increase their autonomy and to separate themselves from the paternalistic relationships that characterized nursing's apprenticeship days, we must remind them that they need to value the supraordinate goal of the institution's fiscal integrity or they will lose an essential laboratory for nursing practice. We have to share the burden of cost containment and teach our students to do the same. Case-mixed, prospective reimbursement is here to stay—in one form or another. It is incumbent on us to prepare ourselves and our future nurses for it. We are challenged to produce an expert clinician with assertiveness and financial and marketing skills, as well as knowledge of power, policies, and politics. These are large challenges that will require us to use all our knowledge and creativity.

DRG GLOSSARY

Appeals—Most disputes between hospitals and the federal government about the prospective payment system must be resolved by administrative or judicial appeals. The Provider Reimbursement Review Board hears administrative appeals.

Base year costs—A hospital's average costs for the cost-reporting period ending on or after September 30, 1982, and before September 30, 1983. During the phase-in of prospective payment, part of a hospital's payments will be based on hospital-specific, base year costs.

Budget neutrality—Medicare payments to hospitals in fiscal 1984 and 1985 may not exceed the amount the federal government would have spent for Medicare inpatient services under the cost control limits outlined in the Tax Equity and Fiscal Responsibility Act of 1982 (TEFRA).

Cancer hospitals—Institutions recognized as a comprehensive cancer center or clinical cancer center by the National Institutes of Health as of April 20, 1983. Fifty percent of the hospital's discharges must have a principal diagnosis of neoplastic disease.

Capital-related costs—Includes depreciation expenses, taxes, leases and rentals, the costs of betterments and improvements, costs of minor equipment, insurance expenses on depreciation assets, interest expenses, the capital-related costs of related organizations, and a return on equity for investor-owned providers.

Case mix index—To eliminate any variations in a hospital's base year costs that are attributable to the complexity of cases it treated, the hospital's base year costs are divided by the 1981 fiscal year case mix index. The index is a statistic that represents the costliness of each hospital's mix of cases compared with a national average case mix.

Diagnosis-related groups of illnesses—Each discharge is classified according to one of 467 DRGs. The DRG system classifies patients into groups that are clinically coherent and homogeneous with respect to resource use.

DRG cost weight—The number, or weight, that reflects a DRG's resource utilization. This weight is multiplied by the average cost for a Medicare discharge to arrive at the payment for the particular DRG.

DRG creep—The practice of manipulating patients' medical record data to upgrade a DRG to a more profitable DRG.

DRGs 468, 469, 470—These DRGs don't group illnesses but are used for administrative purposes.

Direct medical education costs—The costs of approved medical education programs operated directly by the hospital, which will be excluded from the prospective payment system.

Excluded providers—Facilities excluded from prospective payment include alcohol and drug treatment, psychiatric, and rehabilitative hospitals and units, as well as children's and long-term care hospitals and hospitals in states which have alternative payment programs for Medicare.

Grouper—This computer software program screens information from the inpatient bill to assign the DRG. The criteria include patient's age, sex, principal diagnosis, secondary diagnosis, procedures performed, and discharge status.

Indirect medical education costs—Include the additional tests and procedures that residents might order. Payment is based on the number of interns and residents employed at a hospital.

ICD-9-CM—Hospitals code all diagnostic and surgical procedures according to the International Classification of Diseases, 9th Revision, Clinical Modifications, the same code used for DRGs.

Major diagnostic categories—DRGs fall into 23 MDCs. Each MDC corresponds to a single organ system or a combination of an organ system and disease etiology.

Medical review entities—Fiscal intermediaries and peer review organizations will review all inpatient hospital admissions to determine the medical necessity, appropriateness, and quality of care as well as validate the DRG classification.

National rate—The average national costs of treating a Medicare patient, expressed as an urban and rural average and divided into labor- and non-labor-related portions.

Outliers—Cases involving unusually long hospital stays, called day outliers, or unusually costly cases, called cost outliers, gain additional payments to hospitals.

Pass-through costs—Capital-related costs and direct medical education costs, which will be reimbursed on a cost basis until the federal government devises a formula to include reimbursement for these expenditures in prospective payment.

Ping Ponging—A form of gaming to maximize payment, where a patient is transferred back and forth from a hospital or unit participating in prospective payment to an excluded hospital or unit.

Principal diagnosis—The diagnosis that is found to be chiefly responsible for the patient's hospitalization.

Prospective payment—Medicare will pay hospitals a fixed price per discharge for each diagnosis-related group of illnesses.

Prospective payment assessment (PRO PAC)—This independent advisory group will suggest changes in DRG payment rates to the Department of Health and Human Services and recommend changes in the DRG classification system and changes in the DRG cost weights.

Referral centers—Rural hospitals with 500 or more beds will have their rates adjusted by the urban regional and national rates rather than the rural rate. Hospitals must meet certain criteria to qualify as a referral hospital, although the Health Care Financing Administration hasn't yet decided what the adjustment rate will be. Hospitals must admit 50% of their Medicare patients as referrals from other hospitals or by referral from physicians not on the hospital's medical staff. Also, at least 60% of their Medicare patients must live more than 25 miles from the hospital and 60% of all services provided to Medicare patients must be furnished to beneficiaries who live more than 25 miles from the hospital.

Regional rate—The average cost of treating a Medicare patient in each of the nine census divisions. In each region, urban and rural rates are determined, each with labor- and non-labor-related portions. The average regional rate is adjusted to reflect a hospital's wage index, outliers, and the DRG weight.

Sole community hospitals—To qualify as a sole community hospital, a facility must meet any of four criteria: (1) no other hospital is within a 50-mile radius; (2) no other hospital is within a 25- to 50-mile radius and no more than 25% of the residents in its service area use another hospital or no other hospital is accessible, because of weather conditions or geography, for more than one month a year; (3) no other hospital is within 15 to 20 miles away and weather conditions or geography make other hospitals inaccessible for more than one month a year; and (4) it has fewer than 50 beds and no other hospital is within a 25- to 50-mile radius.

Transfer—A patient is considered a transfer when he or she is moved from one unit of the hospital to another; is transferred to another hospital receiving prospective payments; is transferred to a hospital that's in a waived state; or is transferred to a hospital that hasn't yet switched to prospective payment.

Trim points—The average range of the length of stay for a given diagnosis. Diagnoses falling outside the trim points are outliers.

Unbundling—The practice of billing under Part B of the Medicare program for non-physician services provided to a hospital inpatient. Hospitals are now prohibited from unbundling. One exception to the unbundling provision is that physicians can continue to bill Part B for services provided by certified registered nurse anesthetists.

Updating factor—A percentage increase in the hospital market basket for goods and services plus 1%, this factor is applied to a hospital's base year costs for fiscal 1984 and 1985, after adjustment for budget neutrality.

Wage index—The labor-related portion of a hospital's federal payment rates are multiplied by an urban or rural wage index that represents local hospital wages in the metropolitan statistical area within which a hospital is located.

BIBLIOGRAPHY

American Hospital Association. "Medicare Payment: Special Report 3, Legislative Summary and Management Implication." *Healthcare Financial Management,* 13:8:47-52, August 1983.

Ball, M. J., and T. M. Boyle. "Hospital Information Systems: Past, Present, and Future." *Hospital Financial Management,* February 1980, pp. 12-14.

Bentley, J. D., and P. Butler. "Case Mix Reimbursement: Measures, Applications, Experiments." *Hospital Financial Management,* 3:14, 1980.

––––––– . "Measurement of Case Mix." *Topics in Health Care Financing,* 8:4:1-12, 1982.

Bisbee, G., and H. Bachofer. "Usefulness of Case Mix Systems as a Tool in Hospital Management Must Be Determined." *Hospital Services Research,* 2:2:28-31, 1979.

Boerma, Hans. *DRG Evaluation Volume IV-B: The Organizational Impact of DRGs.* Princeton, NJ; Health Research and Educational Trust of New Jersey at the Center for Health Affairs, 1983.

Caterinicchio, R., and J. Warren, "DRGs and Medical Practice: Meeting the Challenge of Incentive Reimbursement." *The Journal of the Medical Society of New Jersey,* 1982, pp. 895-898.

Connor, R. "Case-based Payment Systems: Eight Indicators to Watch." *Hospital & Health Services Administration,* 27:43, 1982.

Curtin, L. L. "Determining Costs of Nursing Services Per DRG." *Nursing Management,* April 1983, pp. 16-20.

Davis, C. "The Federal Role in Changing Health Care Financing." *Nursing Economics,* September-October 1983, p. 104.

Dowling, W. L. "Prospective Rate Setting: Concept and Practice." *Topics in Health Care Financing,* 3:2:8, 1979.

Evans, R. G. " 'Behavioral' Cost Functions for Hospitals." *Canadian Journal of Economics,* 4:2:198-215, 1971.

Ewell, C. "A Look at How New Jersey's DRG System Is Changing Board Roles." *Trustee,* January 1984, pp. 24-29.

Fedorowicz, J., and S. Veazie. "Automated DRG Systems: Unanswered Questions." *Hospital Progress,* 62:1:54-55, 71, January 1981.

Feldstein, M. S. "Hospital Cost Variations and Case Mix Differences." *Medical Care,* 3:2:95-103, 1965.

Fetter, R. B., Y. Chin, J. Freeman, R. Averill, and J. Thompson. "Case Mix Definition by Diagnosis-Related Groups." *Medical Care,* 18:2:12, 1980.

Goldstein, J. R. "Lessons from the New Jersey Experience: From the Top Down." *Health Care Strategic Management,* October 1983, p. 18.

_____ . *Summary of Public Comments and Departments Responses Re. N.J.A.C. 8:31B-3.19 Implementation of RIM Methodology.* Trenton, NJ: State of New Jersey Department of Health, July 19, 1982.

Gonnella, J. S., D. Z. Louis, and J. J. McCord. "The Staging Concept—An Approach to the Assessment of Outcome of Ambulatory Care." *Medical Care,* 14:1:13-21, 1976.

Goodisman, L. D., and T. Trompeter. "Hospital Case Mix and Average Charge per Case: An Initial Study." *Health Services Research,* 14:1:44-55, 1971.

Grimaldi, P. "Equity and Efficiency Implications of Case Mix Reimbursements in New Jersey." In *Profiles of Medical Practice, 1980,* edited by G. L. Glandon and R. J. Shapiro. Chicago: American Medical Association, 1980.

Halloran, E. J. and M. Kiley. "Case Mix Management." *Nursing Management,* February 1984, pp. 39-45.

Health Care Financing Administration. *The National Hospital Rate-Setting Study: A Comparative Review of Nine Prospective Rate-Setting Programs.* Washington, DC: Health Care Financing Administration, Office of Research, Demonstration, and Statistics, 1980.

_____ . *Prospective Payment Provisions: Title VI of the Social Security Amendments of 1983 (P.L. 98-21).* Washington, DC: Government Printing Office, 1983.

Hospital Financial Management Association. *Data Processing Information Survey: Chicago Area Hospitals.* Oak Brook, IL; HFMA, First Illinois Chapter, 1981.

"How Can Hospitals Respond to Medicine Payment Changes?" *Trustee,* December 1983, pp. 18-23.

Jacobs, S. E. "Hospital-wide Computer Systems: The Market and the Vendors," *MUG Quarterly,* 12:3:1-12, Fall 1982.

Jelinek, R., and F. Pierce. "A Nursing System Approach: Productivity and Quality of Care." *Public Productivity Review,* September 1983, p. 223.

Joel, L. "Case Mix Reimbursement: DRGs, RIMs." *The Massachusetts Nurse,* January 1983, pp. 5-6.

————— . "DRG's and RIM's: Implications for Nursing," *Nursing Outlook,* January/February 1984, pp. 42-49.

Lave, J. R., and L. B. Lave. "The Extent of Role Differentiation among Hospitals," *Health Services Research,* 6:15-38, 1971.

Lave, J. R., and S. Leinhardt. "The Cost and Length of a Hospital Stay." *Inquiry,* 13:327-343, 1976.

Maher, A. B., and B. Dolan. "Determining Costs of Nursing Services." *Nursing Management,* September 1982, p. 17.

Morrison, P. G., and R. Caterinicchio. "Case Mix Project." *New Jersey Nurse,* September/October 1980, pp. 1, 7, 10.

Naisbitt, J. *Megatrends.* New York: Warner Books, Inc., 1982.

New Jersey Department of Health. *A Prospective Reimbursement System Based on Patient Case Mix for New Jersey Hospitals, 1976-1983.* Second Annual Report, Vol. 1. Trenton, NJ: State of New Jersey Department of Health, December 1978.

————— . *A Prospective Reimbursement System Based on Patient Case Mix for New Jersey Hospitals, 1976-1983: Case Mix Performance Study, Instruction Manual.* Trenton, NJ: State of New Jersey Department of Health, September 1979.

Nursing and Nursing Education: Public Policies and Private Actions. Washington, DC: National Academy Press, 1983.

Piper, L. P. "Accounting for Nursing Function in DRGs." *Nursing Management,* 14:11:46-48, November 1983.

Plomann, M. *Nine Patient Classification Schemes: Development, Description, and Testing.* Chicago: Health Research and Educational Trust, 1982.

Powell, P. "Fee-for-Service." *Nursing Management,* 14:3:13-19, 1983.

Robinson, M. L. "Special Report: HCFA's Computerized PPS." *Prospective Payment Guide,* 1:3:5, November 1983. U.S. Government Printing Office.

Spitzer, Roxanne B. "Legislation and New Regulations." *Nursing Management,* February 1983.

The Tax Equity and Fiscal Responsibility Act of 1982: Provisions Affecting the Medicare and Medicaid Programs (P.L. 97-248). New York: Ernst & Whinney, 1982.

Toffler, A. *Previews and Premises.* New York: William Morrow and Co., Inc., 1983.

Ullman, R., and G. F. Kominski. "Hospital Reimbursement in the State of New Jersey." Unpublished case study (1981) available from the Sloan Foundation.

White Paper on the Relative Intensity Measures (RIMs) Methodology Developed by the New Jersey State Department of Health to Incorporate Measures of Nursing Intensity into the Diagnosis-Related Group (DRG) Prospective Payment Mechanism. New York: Deloitte, Haskins and Sells, January 1983.

ABOUT THE AUTHORS

Sonja P. Bennett, RRA (registered records administrator), is director of medical records at Riverview Medical Center in Red Bank, NJ.

Carolyne K. Davis, RN, PhD, is administrator of the Health Care Financing Administration, Washington, DC.

Jane Fedorowicz, PhD, is assistant professor of accounting and information systems at the J.J. Kellogg Graduate School of Management at Northwestern University, Evanston, IL.

James M. Gaynor, Jr., is a partner in McDermott, Will, & Emery, a Chicago-based law firm with offices in Boston, Miami, Springfield, and Washington, DC. Mr. Gaynor is in the health law department.

Jane Meier Hamilton, RN, MSN, is a nursing consultant in the metropolitan Philadelphia area.

Ruth Hanft is a health policy consultant in Washington, DC.

Lucille A. Joel, RN, EdD, FAAN, is professor and director of clinical affairs and director of the Teaching Nursing Home Project at the Rutgers University College of Nursing in New Brunswick, NJ.

Dean A. Kant is an attorney in the health law department of McDermott, Will & Emery, a Chicago-based law firm with offices in Boston, Miami, Springfield, and Washington, DC.

157

Pamela J. Maraldo, RN, PhD, is executive director of the National League for Nursing, New York, NY.

Elizabeth M. Mills is a third-year law student at Northwestern University in Evanston, IL.

Marilyn Peacock Plomann, MM, is assistant director of the Hospital Research and Educational Trust, the research and development affiliate of the American Hospital Association, Chicago, IL. She is also project director for the Plannng, Budgeting, and Clinical Management Systems Project being conducted at Hospital Research and Educational Trust.

Susan C. Reinhard, RN, MSN, is lobbyist for the New Jersey State Nurses Association. She also is an instructor of nursing at the College of Nursing of Rutgers—The State University in Newark, and works in addition as a per-diem staff nurse at the Hunterdon Medical Center, Flemington, NJ.

Franklin A. Shaffer, RN, EdD, is deputy director for operations at the National League for Nursing, New York, NY.

Sara E. Smith, RN, MSN, is associate director of nursing education at Ohio Valley General Hospital School of Nursing in Wheeling, WV.

Rosalinda M. Toth, RN, MS, is director of the Department of Nursing and assistant hospital director at the Newark Beth Israel Medical Center in Newark, NJ.